DEFEATING DEMENTIA

FRANCIS C. MCNEAR

Be sure to visit our website,

DefeatingDementiaSMA.com

for news on dementia and

dementia studies.

If you have questions or would like to be added to our email list to receive information on new developments, please contact info@defeatingdementiasma.com

ISBN-13: 978-1-7901-3376-5

DEDICATION

For my wife, Patricia,

who stuck with me through it all.

CONTENTS

ACKNOWLEDGMENTS

This manuscript, that started out as *Descent into Dementia*, a morbid tale of losing my mind, and morphed into the book you are reading, has been seven years in the making.

I will forever be grateful to my wife Patricia for her patience, love and support, especially when I could barely take care of myself.

I would be remiss if I failed to express my gratitude for my son Matthew. There were times in the beginning when suicide appeared to be a solution. His constant support and encouragement always kept me from giving in to despair, never allowing the idea to become an option.

Dr. Dale Bredesen will always be my personal hero and savior. Without his work and encouragement, I would not have the life I enjoy today. He will always have my profoundest gratitude.

I would like to thank Thom Mount, who when I got off track with the protocol and experienced returning cognitive decline, assured me I could regain lost ground if I persevered.

I also want to express my gratitude to India Taylor. Her editing was a godsend and the knowledge of elder care and dementia she contributed made for a better book. Her belief in the project was invaluable.

PROLOGUE

Do you hear yourself or someone you love saying the words, "I can't remember" or “I don't remember” more frequently? Are you wondering if something seriously wrong may be starting to happen? Afraid to find out? Don’t really want to know what’s going on? YOU ARE NOT ALONE. That was me about seven years ago. By keeping things to myself and not getting any type of professional care for several years, I almost lost not only my mind but everything I owned. Thanks to a recent breakthrough in dementia studies and treatment, today I am recovering from Early Onset Alzheimer’s. That is correct. I am one of thousands of people in the United States following the recently developed Bredesen Protocol, and as a result, my memory and my life are being restored to order.

There are hundreds of books that have been written about dementia. There are none, however, that have been written by someone who went through it and eventually found a solution. Prior to Dr. Dale Bredesen's recently published book, *The End of Alzheimer's*, I had not encountered any that have presented real hope. That is because until very recently there was no hope. Alzheimer's, and most other forms of dementia, has always been considered progressive, fatal and incurable.

That is simply no longer the case. People today are recovering. I am one of them. I have met and spoken to others. I have also met Dr. Bredesen, the man who with his team of researchers at UCLA and The Buck Institute in Marin County, California, made these recoveries possible, recoveries that until now did not exist. As that same highly regarded doctor has said, "We are living in the dawn of the Age of Reversible Alzheimer's."

In 2009, I began having serious problems with my memory. By 2012, I had been diagnosed with Early Onset Alzheimer's and my life was literally falling apart. I spent years living with fear and depression. I practically destroyed my finances through countless errors in my business and investments, severely compromising my family's financial future in the process. In 2014, almost broke and certain I would die within a few years, my wife and I moved to Mexico.

Later that year I learned of a treatment protocol for dementia that was having extraordinary success in reversing the symptoms of Alzheimer's. Eventually, I met the man responsible for its creation and began earnestly following the protocol as I understood it at that time. Within months, my mind and my life started improving significantly. I am going to share with you the details of my descent into dementia and my subsequent ongoing recovery from it. My journey has been one that until now had no return passage. It was always a one-way trip. The good news of this book is that this is no longer true.

There are thousands of people following this protocol today and 80 percent of them are experiencing the same life-saving results that I am. In the few years since I met Dr. Bredesen, he has continued to learn more about Alzheimer’s and has continued to refine his protocol, a treatment plan he now prefers to call ReCODE (Reversing Cognitive Decline). In my mind, it will always be the Bredesen Protocol. To see and talk to the people practicing his program you would never guess they had ever suffered from dementia. The last two doctors I visited said basically the same thing about me.

There is a new case of Alzheimer's appearing every six or seven seconds. People are afraid and desperate for information. Almost every day there is another article about a “breakthrough” in the search for a cure and these headlines sell lots of newspapers and magazines.

Unfortunately, while at a glance they seem so encouraging, the stories are often about studies that are years away from being available to humans. Others are based on theories and some merely present speculation.

Prior to the recent publication of Dr. Bredesen’s *The End of Alzheimer’s*, no one had come out and said, "We are reversing the symptoms of dementia" or even, "We have succeeded in halting the progression of the disease."

Today many people, including myself, are saying exactly that.

If you can relate to a life that is suddenly beset with a whole host of problems that are the result of recurring incidents of memory loss, this book is for you. If you have suddenly found yourself full of memory-related fear, sadness, and depression, or if you are caring for a person in that situation, in these pages you will find HOPE and a way out.

Dementia does not announce itself. Rather, it enters your life like a thief in the night. A day at a time, a week at a time, an incident at a time, it slowly steals your life. No one wants to admit they might be losing their mind; the thought is too painful. And so, we remain silent.

The faster you face your problem; just that much faster will you recover. My intention is to provide you with information that will help you and the people who love you successfully cope with dementia.

INTRODUCTION

Before my diagnosis of Early Onset Alzheimer's, when my problems had first begun, I refused to believe there was anything seriously wrong. I did not know I had a disease.

Dementia did not descend on me full-blown. The progression was slow and subtle. It entered my life very gradually, and it was years before I knew, or was willing to admit I knew, that it was there. When dementia begins to start its work, it is actually invisible. It is a process that can take as many as a dozen years, occasionally longer, to complete.

Eventually, I could no longer hide it from myself. In fact, I became certain that I had Alzheimer's Disease. I knew very little about it, but I was sure I had it. I was totally unaware that there were many other types of cognitive impairment, and that some have always been considered to be reversible. I believed it was always fatal and I was doomed. So, I carried on as the wreckage around me continued to mount, and the disease continued to progress.

My recollections of 2010 through 2013 are mostly a blur. I do know that in 2012 I started taking Aricept, a medication for Alzheimer's. I was one of the lucky ones for whom the medicine made a significant difference. Unfortunately, much damage had already been done to my life and relationships, and though it helped, I was still having major problems.

In 2014, having sold our home at a fire sale price, we moved to Mexico where I expected to die within a few years. It was later that year I learned of Dr. Bredesen and the success he was having in reversing the symptoms of Alzheimer's. In May of 2015, I met with him at his lab in California and began following his protocol in earnest, as I understood it at that time.

Within months things started to improve. I began to feel physically better than I had in years and my memory was improving as well. Suddenly, for the first time in what seemed like forever, I was feeling hope. In the time since then, hope has changed to belief.

My wish today is that my readers will be able to avoid much of the damage I created by trying so hard to hide my problem and waiting so long to seek help and instead find the recovery I am enjoying. I am going to show you exactly how to do that.

I am certain I would have experienced a very different outcome if I had not been so concerned with hiding my problem. But how do you go to your partner, to your

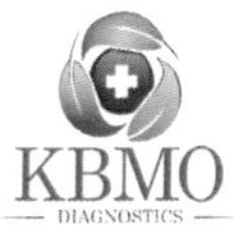

COVID-19 Instructions: Fingerstick Collection, Shipping and Reporting

COVID-19 Test Instructions

1	Wash hands. Continue to run hand under warm/hot water and massage to create blood flow. Make sure you are hydrated; drink water 10-20 minutes prior to sample collection.
2	Clean the site with the provided alcohol swab and allow to air dry.
3	Use the side of the fingertip on either the middle or ring finger. Do not use the center pad of the finger - it is the most sensitive area.
4	Position the lancet provided over the sterilized area and press firmly against your fingertip. Discard the lancet after use. Gently massage your hand moving towards the puncture site to create blood droplets.
5	Fill each circle on the provided collection card with blood. It is important to *completely fill each circle* to ensure enough sample can be obtained to properly administer the test. ****At least 3 spots must be filled to run the panel.**
6	Label the collection card with name and date of collection. Wait 20 minutes until the blood has dried completely on the card before placing it inside the provided biohazard bag, sealing it and placing it inside the provided return envelope.
7	Ship the sample and completed requisition form in the provided return packaging. (Shipping pak with prepaid label or pre-stamped envelope) to: KBMO Diagnostics 4 Business Way Hopedale, MA 01747
8	KBMO Diagnostics will analyze the sample and send the report to the provider 48-72 hours *after the receipt* of the sample.

For instructions please watch this short video at the link below:
https://kbmodiagnostics.com/bloodspot-tutorial-video/

<u>For general support/ questions please contact the lab</u>:

Phone: 617-933-8130
Email: Info@KBMODiagnostics.com
Website: www.KBMODiagnostics.com

Acceptable Blood Spots
Vs.
Unacceptable Blood Spots

Instructions:

Acceptable Sample: Below is an example of the blood spots required for using this test, with three circles completely filled. Once completed, your blood spots should match as closely as possible to the image below.

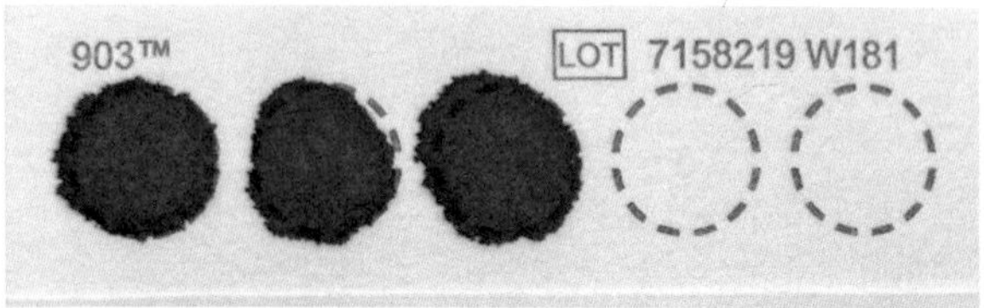

Unacceptable Sample: Below is an example of an unacceptable blood spot card. If the circles are not completely filled, then we do not have enough blood to run the test. A sample that looks like this would be rejected, and a new sample would need to be sent in.

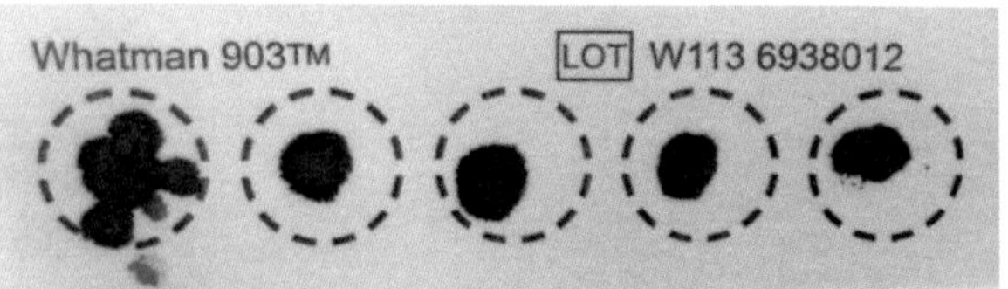

For instructions please watch this short video at the link below
https://kbmodiagnostics.com/bloodspot-tutorial-video/

boss, coworkers or even your friends, and say, "I think I am losing my mind?" I was not willing to do that, and I suspect most other people are not either.

Four years ago, it would have been impossible for me to write this book. I did not have the mental acuity to do so. There were days when it was difficult for me to complete a sentence. That is no longer the case. The people I know today have no idea I have dementia unless I tell them. I am not 100 percent recovered; I still have days when I am forgetful, but that is normal for people of my age. As I write this, I am 68 years old. The difference between my life now and my life five years ago is the difference between night and day, darkness and light.

I no longer wake up depressed and fearful, constantly worrying about what I may have forgotten, or what may come out of my mouth. I am no longer afraid to socialize. I've stopped hoping to die before my life insurance policy expires. Gone is the constant stress of struggling to appear normal. Instead, I wake up each morning grateful to be alive and excited about what the day may bring. I have plans for the future and every reason to believe they will materialize. These changes seem miraculous to me, yet they are based on the science Dr. Bredesen introduced to the world. And based on my experience, I honestly believe they can happen for you too.

Godspeed on your journey.

WHAT IT WAS LIKE

I don’t remember exactly when I started to realize I had above average intelligence. I wasn't a genius, that's for sure, but I was bright. I was told by two high school principals that I had a very high IQ.

I started reading at a very young age, devouring anything I could get my hands on. I read every single Hardy Boys book, one after the other, and when I was through, I even read all of my sister's Nancy Drew books.

Throughout my adult life, I used my intellect to succeed in almost any endeavor I tried. Lawyers talk about the “smartest person in the room.” I didn’t hear that expression until I was in my fifties, but when I did, it was a colleague saying that many times it applied to me. And I had to admit that I thought he was probably right. I realize this may sound arrogant and boastful. I am not bragging, I simply want you to know at what level my brain functioned before my problems began.

I recognized that my brain was my most important asset. So, I believed that with it I would never have too much to worry about, I would always be able to take care of me and mine. I had no idea how mistaken I was.

At the age of 52, I was the Executive Director of a 501c3, a not-for-profit company, with dozens of employees in two countries and as many states. I was ultimately responsible for a budget of millions of dollars. I had a beautiful home in New England and another in the Caribbean. I had a decent retirement account, savings investments and a fund for my son's education. Little did I know that less than ten years later I would be unable to supervise even one employee, let alone seventy. It never occurred to me that not only would my cognitive abilities erode, but that almost all my other assets would fade away right along with them.

By the time things started to get really problematic, I had been back in the Caribbean for several years. I had left there in 2000 to get my Master's degree and to work with troubled children. It had been a semi-retirement but seven years later I was back in the islands. My wife would have much preferred to stay in New England, but my retirement had been financially premature, so once again she packed everything up and home we went.

Our house had been on the executive rental market for seven years by the time we returned. It had provided a nice income during that period, but the four separate tenants had taken a toll on the house and the grounds. There was a lot of restoration to be done, inside and out: new plants to be bought and planted, furniture to be replaced or reupholstered, rooms to be painted. It was a busy period, and between working on the house and reconnecting with old friends, it was a happy period as well. In New England, I had been constantly involved with work. I felt like I was also reconnecting with my wife, and it felt good.

I was very happy to be back. St. Croix was the first place I had ever really felt like a part of a community, at home. And it is a great place to be able to call home. The island is incredibly diversified, with Arabs, West Indians and people of Spanish descent coexisting with an adventurous breed of Americans and a sprinkling of Danes to further spice up the pot.

St. Croix, like everywhere, has problems, but when we were there I felt like a part of the solution. My company had employed dozens and dozens of young men over the years and we were good corporate citizens. A few years ago, while visiting the island, a young man of forty told me that working for my company had been the best job he ever had. I felt like I knew everyone, and everyone knew me. It was a good feeling.

Our son, who was raised there, is to this day is an amazing young man. I am certain that growing up color blind, sharing a crib for several years with a delightful young boy, a boy of a different race, who is now a Captain in the United States Air Force, played a big role in that. They share a strong bond to this day.

We were living in a house that we had designed for ourselves. It was my favorite house on the island. I had always thought I would finish my life in the Caribbean, that hopefully when the time came, I would die at home in my mahogany four-poster bed. But I certainly had no intention of doing that anytime soon.

We practically lived on the gallery, which was almost as big as the house. It had huge potted palms, a teak table and chairs, rocking chairs, old Oriental rugs, a built-in couch and, of course, a hammock. And, there was also an area for grilling from which the aroma of sizzling steaks was a regular occurrence. A few short steps took you down to the pool and hot tub as well as a small basketball court where I had taught my son the art of the three-point shot.

The house was high on a hill, looking down on the town, the harbor to the left and the south shore to the right. The view was among the best on the island. Boats going in and out of the harbor day and night, and other islands on the horizon, provided an ever-changing scene. We were in one of the very best neighborhoods. We loved it. It had never occurred to me that five years later we would have to rent it and take up residence in an 800-square foot tract house. Eventually, we were forced to sell our home. It was painful, but dementia left us no choice. Dementia made many decisions for us, several I was not even aware of.

We got to enjoy our home without incident for about three years. Then things started to change. The change occurred slowly, subtly. At the beginning, the bumps in the road were infrequent. I think I was aware of most of them, but I am not sure of that, and I didn't really worry about it too much. My employees began telling me I needed "memory powder." I told myself that for far too long.

When I first admitted to myself that something was seriously wrong, my mind went immediately to Alzheimer's. I didn't even know how to spell it, but I was sure I had it. I knew absolutely nothing about dementia. I had no idea there were any different types of cognitive impairment, some reversible and some not fatal. All I knew about was Alzheimer's, and I knew almost nothing about that other than it would kill you. Unfortunately, the brain does not know what it does not know. As it turns out, I was even wrong about the “fact” that it always killed you.

Because I didn't want anyone to know I had this awful disease, I did everything I could do to conceal my condition from family, friends, and coworkers until it was impossible to do so. I think I even tried to hide it from myself. I believe that when I started to think I was literally losing my mind, it was simply too painful to deal with. So, like many others before me, I tried to deny it.

Also, because I believed there was no cure for what I had, I delayed seeking medical attention way too long. As a result of my own experience, I can say with certainty, "DEAL WITH IT. THE SOONER THE BETTER!"

Had myself and my wife been fully aware of what was happening, I believe the last six years of my life would have gone very differently. Unfortunately, when you are forgetting things, you are not aware of what you are forgetting. Nor are you aware of the things you are not attending to.

If she had known exactly what was occurring, my wife would have paid much more attention to our finances. As it was, I had always been, and continued to be, in charge of all things related to money. Managing savings and investments was my responsibility. When she did start to notice that things were not quite right, I only became defensive. Huge mistake.

I owned what had once been a large and successful painting company in the Virgin Islands. The company did an equal mix of residential, commercial and government contracts, everything from multi-million-dollar homes to schools, hospitals and public housing projects. One of my roles in the business was to be the estimator. Up until then, I had been very good at it. It was one of the reasons we were prosperous.

Unfortunately, when I had originally reopened my painting business, not only did I not know I was suffering from the beginnings of dementia, I also didn't know that one of the defining symptoms of dementia is an inability to plan and execute complex projects, or correctly estimate the time it will take to complete them. So, I kept on estimating, and these were large projects. I was estimating the time, materials and manpower it would take to paint hospitals, schools, airport additions and one-hundred-unit condominium complexes. I was also unaware that my previously excellent math skills were rapidly deteriorating. It was a perfect stage for disaster. Part of me knew that I was not making any money, but I had no idea why. Denial was keeping me from learning the truth, not only about my health but the company's health as well. By 2011, I was incapable of doing any real accounting. My wife, however, was painfully aware that I was operating the business on money I was borrowing from our personal resources, which were steadily depleting.

Another reason I had been successful was that I had always maintained very good relations with all my clients. Builders, government officials and homeowners all knew they could count on me to be honest and to do what I said I would. The Virgin Islands are like that. Reliability is at such a premium that if you just show up on time and do what you promise, and do it right, more business will usually follow. And, if you do it well, return business is a guarantee. God removes paint in the Caribbean at about twice the speed that he does in the rest of the world.

Eventually, I began to admit to myself that things were getting bad. The following notes, taken in July 2011, will give you an idea of how bad. They are presented in the exact way that I wrote them, and they represent the beginning of the breakdown of my denial system.

A guy gave me a check for some consulting work about a month ago. I found it yesterday. I had never deposited it, in fact I had forgotten that I even had it. Later that day I remembered that I had forgotten to bill my last client. That had been about a month ago too. A few day ago I stopped to get gas and tried to pump it from the nozzle that was still hooked up to the pump. At least nobody saw that. A month ago at the same station I went in, paid for my gas, went out and drove away without pumping the gas. Everybody said that was no big deal, just part of growing older. Then I did it again. I was willing to accept that I was aware of all of those things. Wonder what happened that I wasn't aware of? That's a scary thought.

My biggest fear is that I won't remember my family, and it will break their hearts. They say I won't even be aware of it. And they say that people with the disease get nasty. I am mean enough already.

These notes were written at a time when I had told no one other than my wife that I might have a problem. It's interesting to me that I seemed to remember everything as having happened "about a month ago." I was clearly losing the ability to keep track of time. It was also around this time I started driving right past job sites when I was delivering supplies to them. More than once, I found sets of blueprints in my office that had mistakenly been set aside and forgotten about. These were plans for projects I had been asked to bid on. They represented builders that no doubt had asked themselves, "What's up with him?"

For many years, I was in the habit of meeting a group of friends at a restaurant on the waterfront for Sunday brunch. The restaurant was located on the boardwalk at the end of a large shopping arcade. One day, as I walked past the arcade, I suddenly recalled that six or seven weeks earlier (who knows, it may have been longer) I had met with the arcade's manager. We had toured the property and I had promised her an estimate for a painting contract by the end of the week. It was a job I had done once before, about 9 years previously, and it would be an easy proposal to prepare. I had walked from that meeting and not given it another thought until that morning I walked past it, almost two months later. Usually, on these Sunday mornings, I parked next to the restaurant. That day there were no spaces, so I parked a few blocks away. Had I not had to walk by the arcade to meet my friends I may never have remembered. I tried contacting her the next day with an excuse, but it was too late. A sixty or seventy thousand-dollar contract had slipped through my fingers, along with another part of my reputation for reliability.

My father had once told me, “Don’t make customers out of your friends, make friends out of your customers.” I had always been a people person and made friends quickly. I was also genuinely interested in making sure my customers got more than they were expecting. I viewed my business as an opportunity to serve not only my customers but my employees as well.

As my memory worsened, there were a lot of changes in the way I interacted with people. I became anxious and tried to have as little contact with my customers as possible. And, when we did interact, it was not always pleasant. There were times when I was so unaware of what my employees were doing that I could no longer control the quality of the product they were producing. Near the end, we spent many months working on the remodeling of, and additions to, a small estate that belonged to a good friend's girlfriend. It was a beautiful property she had just bought, and she was enjoying the process of creating a space that was just right for her and her many guests. I had a painter on the job who had been trained in Europe and who, ten years earlier, I had believed was one of my best employees. I still did. He was my foreman on the job, the one that was supposed to make sure things went right.

One day, I was standing in the yard talking with the homeowner, a very pleasant woman. It was eight o'clock on another perfect day in the Caribbean. We were admiring the view when this particular painter pulled into the driveway. I was shocked when she said, " I cringe every time I see him coming."

"Why is that, has he said something to offend you?", I inquired.

"It's not what he says, but what he does. He leaves paint on the floor wherever he goes." I could see she was really distressed.

That was the last thing I thought I would ever hear about him. To make the situation even worse, all the floors were brand new Brazilian Cherry. They were gorgeous. While I was happy that she had finally told me what was happening, the damage had been done. Not to the floors, I could fix that, but to my reputation. I later realized other aspects of my relationship with this customer were not as good as I was accustomed to.

On two occasions, trying to be helpful, I had told this woman less than flattering things about the general contractor she had hired for her remodeling project. I now know that she did not appreciate hearing these remarks from me but at the time I lacked the clarity to pick up on that. She was quite pleased with him at that point and all I was doing was detracting from her enjoyment of the process of renovating her home. This lady had previously done several very large renovations with much success and she was probably rightfully proud of her skill at it. The awareness of the gravity of these incidents only occurred to me in retrospect. Customer relations are a huge part of success for anyone in the business of providing a service.

On an island, whenever you go to any event you are certain to meet people that you know. One Saturday afternoon I went to an art show and while there I ran into this same woman and three of her friends. She introduced me to one of them. I had not noticed that she was the same age as her, and I asked if the friend was her daughter. Don't ask me why. I guess I was trying to make conversation and said the first thing that came out of my mouth. All four ladies were almost speechless. I stopped going to events like that not too much later. St. Croix is a very small island and I knew that I would run into people and not remember their names, and maybe not their faces. I stopped doing a lot of the things I had once enjoyed.

One of the activities in the islands that I really enjoyed was sailing. I had never bought a boat in all the years we were there, but I always had one close friend with a sailboat. During the period I was having problems with my memory, that friend was John. He had a 42-foot Waverly Ketch he loved to sail. Many times, just the two of us sailed to other islands. At least a couple of Sundays a month, he would invite a gang of us to sail out to Buck Island, a small offshore island that was actually a National Park. The beach is pristine, and the water is so clear that you can read your watch 30 feet below the surface. These excursions were always fun and were among the most enjoyable aspects of my great life. The last year I lived on St. Croix I stopped going on these trips because I was embarrassed by how much I had forgotten about sailing. I could no longer even remember how to tie off a cleat.

I really have no idea how many appointments I made and forgot about back then, but I know there were several. There was a hotel on the waterfront that my company had painted about 10 years prior to this period. One of the first things I had noticed when I returned from my sojourn in New England was that it had not been repainted since. And it needed to be.

For over a year I kept telling myself to stop in and speak to the owner. It was the same man I had worked for 10 years previously and he had been very pleased with the work we had done then. I kept forgetting all about it. On more than one occasion I walked by his office and saw that he was in. Instead of knocking on his door and taking care of business, I just walked on by, making sure he didn't see me. Not only was I forgetting, I was now also procrastinating, very unlike my usual way of doing things. I think this was the result of the difficulty I was having in my interactions with others. I was getting more and more uncomfortable in social and business situations alike. I was beginning to live in a constant state of low-level fear. I finally bit the bullet. I went to his office and reintroduced myself.

Of course, he remembered me, and he was, in fact, glad to see me. He had been thinking of repainting the hotel for some time. I told him I would have a quote for him within two weeks and never thought about it again until the day I walked by and saw a crew of painters hard at work. A hotel contract in a highly visible location is not only lucrative, it is also a couple of months of free advertising.

Actually, I had thought about it a few times, but then I would procrastinate until I forgot again. This was totally unlike me. I had always been very aggressive about going after contracts. On one level, I knew something very different was happening, but I honestly didn't give it a great deal of thought. It's hard to give anything much thought when you are constantly forgetting. There was now obviously a different person running my company, a person who was pretty much doomed to failure.

These types of things did not happen every day or even every week. There were periods when I felt like everything was the way it had always been: easy. During these periods I would enjoy life as I always had, and I would forget the strange events that were taking place. I would even get an occasional contract where I actually made money. St. Croix is such an incredibly beautiful place that the ugliness trying to take over my life was having a hard time getting my full attention.

I had then, and I still have now many friends on the island. They are a diverse group of people that come from many walks of life. Several have businesses and all of them are pretty intelligent folks, hoteliers and homemakers, musicians and masseuses, lawyers and landscape architects, to name just a few. And I have known a lot of them for over thirty years. Not one of them really believed I was having serious problems. At the end some of them did, but for several years that was not the case. I was good at hiding my condition from people but on the occasions I tried to be honest about it, I was usually met with, "Oh, we're all getting older," or something similar.

I kept underestimating almost every contract we had. I had always been very good at math and now I was making errors in that department all the time. I would look at an existing building, take measurements and notes, and by the time I sat down to do the estimate I would have forgotten certain aspects of the job. I also found that the notes I was taking were often almost illegible. I would underestimate both the time I would need to complete a project as well as the amount of materials involved. And, of course, I would not make a profit.

I would usually end up the low bidder, get the contract and end up having to borrow money from myself to complete the job, thinking I would make it up on the next one. I never did. The occasional times I would make a profit, I would forget to replace the funds I had withdrawn from my personal accounts. If there was ever a positive balance in the company accounts, it would be borrowed money. I was not completely aware this was happening. The loans somehow made me feel like we were at least breaking even.

If another person had been managing my business back then, it would have been perfectly clear the ship was sinking. I can now recall three separate occasions when every other bidder was more than double my price. One time, the only other bidder was three times my price, and once, on a public housing project, my bid was thrown out for being so low that there was doubt we would be able to complete the project. There were dozens of times when I had no knowledge of what others had bid. I am sure they were no different.

I wasn't always the low bidder. One time I did an estimate for a small condominium complex. The manager was a guy I knew, but not well. When I turned in the proposal, I told him something like this: "I want you to know I am sure we will be the low bidder. Please don't think it is too low. I have painted almost every condominium complex on the island. I know how to benefit from the economies of scale and I know how to do that efficiently."

He wasn't very busy at that moment, and he replied, "Come on into my office, and we can open up the other two bids and see who has the best price right now." Imagine my embarrassment when my quote was more than double that of the other two. Another math error, another 60,000 dollars down the drain. It was another extremely uncomfortable situation and one more blow to my reputation.

I think I was taking medication for my memory at this point, but I am not sure. So much of that time in my life was just a blur. It is difficult to remember in just what sequence many of these events took place. If I hadn't been taking notes, I would have no idea at all.

Maybe you can understand why I delayed getting medical attention for so long and maybe you can't. Looking back, I believe it was a combination of things that made me postpone seeking help. In the beginning, it was denial. Later, when things got worse, it was an unwillingness to deal with what I thought must be a terminal illness. Part of me thought my condition was fatal, so why bother. Another part of me kept hoping it would get better. And of course, I was not fully aware of all the mistakes I was making. I might be attuned to them for a day, or a few hours, but then I would go back into denial and carry on as usual. This happened over and over again, with brief periods of what seemed like business as usual interspersed. Those were probably periods where I just wasn't aware of the damage being done.

On one of my son's trips home from college, he began to notice that things were not so good on the economic front. He asked me why we didn't start to downsize. We had a pool that no one had used in a few years, other than when he was home. The basketball court in the backyard had seen no activity for many years as well. We could have rented the property for several thousand dollars a month, and in fact, we eventually did, years later, but by then we were almost broke. His suggestion had fallen on deaf ears, ears that did not want to hear the truth.

Eventually, I went to a psychiatrist. I should have started with a neurologist, an internist, or my family doctor, but as I said, I knew nothing about dementia. Plus, this doctor was Harvard educated, and I assumed he was my best option. After all, where else would you go when you think you are losing your mind? Also, his office was on a different island, and no one would know that I was seeing him.

It was a 200-dollar seaplane ride to get to his office, and his fee was also hefty. It was another monthly expense that I could have avoided by seeing a doctor on St. Croix. It was another example of faulty reasoning quietly breaking the bank. The first year I was seeing him, I had medical insurance. I cannot explain why, but I never put in a claim for those expenses. There is much I can't explain from those years.

The doctor was confident that I was too young to have Alzheimer's. I kept telling him I did. I kept telling him that because, college and postgraduate educated person that I am, I did not know IT'S NOT ALWAYS ALZHEIMER'S. Nor did I know anything about the disease I was so certain I had.

As I kept reporting increasingly worse symptoms, he started suggesting tests. I had no insurance by that time and was losing so much money I felt I could not afford them. I can now see that it must have been very frustrating for him. I eventually had some blood work done as well as a CT scan. Other than some anemia, they showed nothing that would explain my situation. Today, five years later, that anemia would probably be seen as a red flag for more scrutiny of my blood work.

I am certain that more tests would have been the appropriate thing to do, but by now I was very close to broke. Also, believing my condition was incurable, I was not in a hurry to confirm the diagnosis. I later learned that doctors are in no hurry to do that either. In fact, I now know that almost half of all Alzheimer's patients go to their graves without ever having been diagnosed.

He brought up the possibility of Mild Cognitive Impairment (MCI), a type of cognitive dysfunction I knew nothing about. I did know, however, that nothing about my condition felt mild. And so, I continued to try and make him understand that I had Alzheimer’s. I now know that MCI actually can be quite frightening. There was so much I was yet to learn.

Then one day he mentioned that the very first time I walked in his door, he could tell I was depressed, and that sometimes depression led to dementia. He was right; I had been depressed for a very long time.

Eleven years earlier, I had closed my business in the Caribbean in order to go to school, get a Master's degree, and work with troubled children. A few years later, I became Executive Director of a therapeutic boarding school. When I took the position, I had no idea the school had been embroiled in legal issues for years and that the State wanted to close it down. In fact, they had been trying for years to do just that.

The State wanted to bring the school into compliance with regulations that had not been put into law until relatively recently. They had directed the school to stop some of its behavior management policies, which I did. I sometimes wonder if my thinking was a little impaired even back then. Why did I take a position like that without knowing exactly what I was getting into? I accepted the offer without doing any research at all into the history of the school. It was apparent they were doing great things and that was enough for me. I did no due diligence.

Less than a month after I took the job, a State agency descended on the campus like a SWAT team, and for the next three years, I was in the middle of an enormously expensive, highly contentious, extremely public legal battle. I was in and out of court, I was working 70 and 80-hour weeks, and the school was being financially crippled by legal and consulting fees.

For a year and a half, I managed to keep the school open while it was losing 150,000 dollars every single month. I thought then, and I still do, that the work we were doing was a blessing to many children and their families. I knew the program needed to change several things, but I believed in it, I was proud of the changes we were seeing in the children, and I was confident we could get in compliance with the State's requests and maintain our own compliance with integrity. I was dedicated to the children that were trying to complete the program, and I was committed to their parents as well, several of whom I had become friends with. So, I kept on fighting till the bitter end.

The stress of running a school that is losing five thousand dollars every single day is enormous. It is also depressing. There were several weeks when I didn't know if we would make payroll until the day before it was due. I had given up a very lucrative income to do something that I thought was altruistic and here I was being threatened with contempt of court citations and being accused in open court of neglecting children, an accusation that was reported not only in The Boston Globe but in the local papers as well. It was a lot to handle. I was exhausted all the time (a sign of depression), and I thought more than once of suicide.

I have a good friend who has a Master's degree in

Social Work. He had been working at the school for many years. He told me one day, that I mentioned suicide more than anyone he had ever known. I was in therapy during this entire period. It was a requirement of my position. But there were so many other issues to discuss during those sessions that it never occurred to me to raise the topic of depression, nor did the therapist. I find it interesting that I never considered medication, while at the same time I was working with dozens of kids whose treatment included their use.

Thank God, there was a man on the Board of Directors who, in addition to having a daughter at the school, also became a friend and a major emotional support. He was a very busy lawyer, with 40 other lawyers working for the firm that he alone owned. Still, he took almost every phone call I ever made to him, and as time went by, they became more and more frequent. I will forever be grateful to him.

Unfortunately, the culture of the school was too deeply embedded to change. The school had been in existence for almost 30 years and one staff member had been there since he was a student 20 years prior. To make a long story short, the state had said that we had to change or close, and while we did improve many things, the residential staff would not, or could not, adjust to the new behavior management protocols that were required, and the State eventually froze our admissions, a death blow to any private school.

Sadly, the school eventually closed, and the Board of

Directors decided to start another similar one in Florida. We had been sending kids there for many years to study marine biology. When I look back, I question my judgment in having agreed to be a part of the new school. It was 1500 miles from my home in Massachusetts and my family. My son was in his senior year in high school, and yet, I committed to spending every other week on the campus in Florida. It was definitely not my best thinking.

After the school in New England closed, there was an eighteen-month period of managing the property that was now for sale. This included, among many other administrative tasks, emptying out 14 buildings.

During this period, I was functioning effectively in my responsibilities. I did not even suspect I might have a problem, as no evidence of this had begun yet. It was not an issue. I knew I was starting to occasionally forget little things, but it was nothing out of the ordinary. I just started taking more notes.

I did make one major error at the very end of this period. We were still selling assets in New England and money, as always, was in scarce supply. At a meeting of the Board of Directors, the same Board that was responsible for the school in Florida, I was tasked with making sure the comptroller paid the premium on the Directors and Officers insurance policy. It was not inexpensive. This is the policy that protects members of the Board in the event of a lawsuit. When running a school for troubled kids and their often-troubled parents, the possibility of a lawsuit is ever present. This policy was of paramount importance to everyone on the board, including myself. A few hours after the board meeting, during which this issue first came up, I went to the comptroller's office to discuss this with him and impress upon him the importance of the assignment. He would be the one to write the check, and even though he had attended the meeting himself, I wanted to make sure he knew what was expected. I thought that was the end of it. But a Director's responsibility is not simply to give directives. The onus of execution rested squarely on my shoulders, and I had not followed through.

Several months later we had another Board meeting. When the subject of the insurance policy came up, I was as embarrassed as I have ever been. The comptroller, when asked, said he had not kept the policy current. No real explanation, just no. He had apparently decided it was not a priority for him. Not only was I embarrassed, I lost the confidence of the Board. And, I was now personally exposed to liability.

My friend, the lawyer, who immediately became a former friend, resigned from the Board the next day. In retrospect, I regret the loss of my friend more than I regret having had to operate for a few more months uninsured. This was the first incident however, that I could not ignore. Dropping that ball was something I never would have done. Something was going on. Something bad.

The second incident occurred several months later, at the school in Florida that we were trying to establish. At a therapeutic boarding school, many of the kids do not go home for vacation. On holidays, a certain number of residential staff has to stay on campus. It was just before Christmas, in the late afternoon. All the staff was meeting to determine who would take which weeks off.

A dorm parent, who was also a history teacher, put up his hand and asked for a few extra days off. I was livid, and I told him so. "How dare you ask for more time off? I gave you and your girlfriend an extra week off a few weeks ago so you could take advantage of that chance to visit London. You never even said thank you." I was not in the habit of berating members of the staff, especially this one. He was the head of our brand-new sailing program and was doing a fantastic job. Imagine my astonishment when his jaw dropped, and he said, "Does the name Carnaby Street mean anything to you?"

A bell went off in the back of my head. Upon their return, he had called me while they were still unpacking. Not only had he thanked me, he and his girlfriend had brought me a souvenir from the famous street in London we had talked about before they left. My relationship with that couple was forever ruined and my credibility with the rest of the staff was severely compromised.

Shortly after Christmas, I informed what was left of the board that I was resigning, citing family responsibilities. That was true, but I also no longer trusted myself. They asked me to stay until graduation and I agreed. They decided soon after that the school would be having no more graduations after that one; in fact, it was going to close. The thing I had devoted my life to for the last four years would be no more. I know there was nothing I could have done differently that would have made any difference, but I took it as a personal defeat. It triggered an even deeper depression.

By the time I finally resigned, I had been depressed and occasionally experiencing what doctors call "suicidal ideation" for over two years. Had it not been for my son, I believe I may have followed through on that idea. It was a deep depression that did not go away. It is no surprise to me that I looked depressed the first time I entered the doctor's office in 2010.

He believed there was a strong possibility the depression was playing a role in my memory problems. And so, we began a pharmaceutical treatment for depression that I still follow today, though in much lower doses. Within a few months, I was actually feeling happy some days. I had forgotten what that felt like. But my memory problems continued to progress.

In 2009, I had tried to form a partnership with a young man who had run all my field operations when the business had been much larger. He had been working for me since he was twelve or thirteen and, when I had left for New England, he had started his own small company. He was a very talented painter that could get things done faster than anyone I ever met. And he was also a personable young man. In some ways, he felt like a son to me.

Our first big contract was for 25 or 30 units of public

housing. We did the estimate on the trunk of a car after having looked at only one type of unit. There were four different types. We assumed that the three- and four-bedroom units would have the same number of bathrooms, the same size kitchens and the same size living rooms as the one-bedroom unit we had looked at. And, of course, they did not. What should have been a lucrative contract ended up paying our employees, vendors, and everyone's salary but mine and my new partner, whom I paid with my own money. I believe this project was the first one I borrowed money from myself in order to complete. I had never made that type of estimating mistake before, and I am sure I would not have made this one if I had been thinking clearly.

We had agreed that we would each take three weeks of paid vacation. My partner decided to take his children to a nearby island for one of those weeks. I gave him his week's pay before he left, as well as a one-hundred-dollar bill to get souvenirs for his kids. When he returned to work the following Friday, I gave him a check for the week he had been gone. He gave me a funny look at the time, but I didn't think much of it.

A few days later he asked me when he was going to receive his vacation pay and I told him he had been paid for the week he had been on vacation on the day he came back. He said he knew he had been paid for the week he did not work, but that he was also supposed to receive an additional check, that a vacation check was something you were paid in addition to being paid for the time you did not work. Nothing could persuade him that he was misinformed.

I offered to pay for him to consult a lawyer. I also said that it was our company and that, if we wanted to, there was nothing stopping us from having that policy. It would just be an early draw against profits, and we could both do it.

And then he mentioned a bigger problem. I had been promising him a written contract for months. Over and over, I HAD FORGOTTEN. I had never drawn up a contract. No wonder he didn't trust me. Why should he? Any good partnership has to be built on trust and confidence, and he no longer had either. And so, the partnership ended having lasted only seven months. It was a long time before we could have a civil conversation.

That was two years before things got really bad. And it wasn't just the business front that was suffering. I put my wife through hell for many years.

Here are some additional personal notes written in late 2011 or early 2012, again presented exactly as written.

So, my wife drives a Lexus. We have a tight driveway, as in narrow. I needed to take some picture of the car and show then to a guy who's going to replace the windshield. So I took the picture, then got in my truck on the other side of the driveway.

Backing out ten seconds later I almost crashed into the Lexus, because I forgot it was parked there

I wrote what you just read about two weeks ago. This

evening I was going over what I had written, and I had to reread it because I had no recollection of the incident I was describing.

Eventually, just leaving the house became a major production that required my wife's assistance. First, she would have to help me find my phone. This might take two minutes and it might take ten or even fifteen because it was often in very strange places. Once, I found it in the refrigerator, another time in the dirty clothes hamper. Phone in hand, I would head out the door only to return minutes later, to look for my keys. And go through the same thing all over again. One morning I went out to the driveway and saw that her SUV was parked behind my truck. I would have to move it. I went back inside, got her keys (hers were somehow always in the same place), went back out to the driveway, got into my truck and backed straight into her SUV.

There will come a time in the life of everyone who suffers from dementia when the whole issue of driving will become a serious issue. When and how to deal with that issue will be addressed in the chapter *To the Caregivers*.

I only remember these events because of the notes I was taking. I was sure that I was dying from Alzheimer's, and the notes were for what was to be a morbid memoir titled, *Descent into Dementia*. It wasn't until my memory began to improve, in 2015, that I decided to write this book instead.

Another thing I frequently did before I had started

taking medication, was to leave the house with my pants unzipped and my belt undone. I would like to think I caught myself every time I did it, but when you have cognitive impairment you can never be certain. I may have left the house like that many times and just don't remember.

Part of my job was to make sure my employees always had plenty of ice and water. So, into the store I would go, grab several jugs of water, and pay for them as well as a few bags of ice, which were in the ice machine outside. It was the same story: I would not remember to get the ice out of the machine on my way out. At least with the ice, I would catch the problem as soon as I got to the job site. By the third time I did this at the same store, they started to remind me to take the ice. Sometimes, I would still forget and then be too embarrassed to return to the store.

Speaking of employees, another thing that drained my finances was making some of them loans till payday. If you have an impaired memory, lending money is to be avoided like the plague. In fact, everything that has anything to do with finances needs to be written down and monitored closely, ideally with the help of someone else. I rarely remembered to collect on these short-term loans, and when I tried to, they would often say they had already paid me. I had no idea whether they were telling the truth. I am sure I lost a lot of money that way. One of my employees figured out what was going on long before me and would ask for a loan every week, usually on

Monday or Tuesday, thereby giving me plenty of time to forget.

By now, I had a few employees that were not the cream of the human crop. Whereas ten years prior I had a crew of the best painters on the island, as well as several I had relocated from Florida, I now did not have enough steady work to hire pros. Professional painters work for companies that can guarantee them at least 40 hours a week. I had a ragtag crew with guys coming and going all the time. Previously, I would hire guys and they would stay for years and years. Like with so many things, this was no longer the case.

Finally, there was an incident that provided the straw that broke the camel's back. We were doing all the painting on a new government building that was under construction. I had three guys working and they had run out of joint-compound. The paint store was close by, right down the street.

I hopped in my truck and went and bought the compound. Two minutes later, as I was pulling back into the job site, I said to myself, "Oh, I need to get joint compound." I decided to go to a different store and buy some. My house was on the way to this store, so I decided to stop there and see if I had any in my other truck. I parked, got out of the truck I was in, and headed to the other one. As I went around the back of the truck I was driving, I saw the new container I had just purchased through the back window.

That was it. I wanted to give up; I was riddled with

despair. At my next visit to the doctor, I convinced him to start me on Aricept, a well-known Alzheimer's medicine. For weeks nothing changed other than I began to have horrendous, vivid nightmares, just as the manufacturer had warned I might. The dreams were always the same: I was lost in a strange city and could not find my way home and I would not have my phone or wallet and could not remember any numbers. Often in the dream, I would try to contact my wife, and I would find out she had left me. I would come out of the dream in a cold sweat. I would force myself to stay awake for fear the dream would recur. Often it did, or a different one with the same theme.

It was during this period, before the medicine started working, that I filed a claim for Social Security disability benefits. Not only had I severely injured my back during two separate accidents at work (one a definite result of poor thinking), I could no longer do what I had once been so good at, I could no longer run a business. Filing a claim for disability benefits is a long process, and about five or six weeks into it, the Alzheimer's medication I had been taking began to work. Certainly not perfectly, but well enough that I felt I could try working again.

I withdrew my claim as I felt I did not need it anymore. All was not well, but things were infinitely better than before. Six months later the medicine stopped working, and things were even worse. I increased the dose, and after a few weeks it began to work again, but now the writing was on the wall. I reopened my claim and several months later, after having spent an hour and a half being examined by a doctor the Social Security Administration had hired to investigate my claim, it was granted. His diagnosis was pre-senile dementia, or Early Onset Alzheimer's.

When I had experienced such a good response to the medication, I had felt that it was definitely confirmation that I had the disease, which in some ways made me more depressed. I now know, many years later, that the medicine I was taking sometimes works best for people with other types of dementia.

I wrote these notes sometime in 2012

It seems like things are progressing a lot faster these last few weeks. I have a hard time finishing a sentence without making a mistake. Often I cannot remember the word I am looking for, or I will substitute one inappropriate word for another. I heard myself saying, "This thing weighs a fortune," the other day. I think I am going to have to write faster and take more notes because I can't remember All the things that are happening to me every day. I guess there is a time coming when I won't even be aware of what is happening. That's when I will start to slide farther down. I'm not sure which is worse, the embarrassment or the fear that your mind is starting to betray you. And you don't know what the right response is. Should I get angry at my brain for no longer working properly? My brain and I have been through a lot together. The last time I had an IQ test was 7 years ago. It is easy to do when you work at a school. I scored 144. I believe in high school I tested at 152 or 157....for three and a half years I was paid a handsome salary to put words to paper. I wrote Jingles and Radio copy, and PR releases... Yeah, words came easy to me, and now I can rarely finish a thought or a sentence without some type of error. As I am trying to write this almost every sentence has some error that needs to be changed...

I know people have strokes every day and their brains are injured and don't work the same anymore. But this A thing sneaks up on you, one incident at a time, stretched over years. And everyone gets forgetful as they age and you want to think so much that it's just that. So do your friends and family. They constantly tell you that what is going on around you is normal. But there comes a point where it finally becomes as obvious to them as it is to you. And you get scared; you get petrified, because the disease is horrible... I can't imagine what it's like to look at your only son and not know who he is. So, before you feel that pain now, long before it is actually happening ...

It is a pain too heavy to hold. So, you try to stay in denial. Some days you can, and some days you can't. And then, you just wish you could die now...

Those were the events happening to me and the feelings I was having on a regular basis before I started to get better. The notes accurately convey my constant state of mind in the month preceding our move to Mexico in 2014. When we arrived in Mexico my intention was to live out my remaining days in a small town where I wouldn't get lost and where hopefully my wife would be able to find the care I was surely going to need at an affordable price.

It is three years later now and it is amazing to me just how bad my writing, typing, and punctuation were back then, and how much it has improved. The same is true of my attitude. I no longer wake up with feelings of gloom and doom, dreading to start the day. I have not had those feelings for many months.

San Miguel de Allende is a magical small city in the mountains of central Mexico, about three hours north of Mexico City. I visited it for the first time when I was 20 years old when it was a much smaller town. I fell in love with it then, and I still love it today. Over the years it has transformed into quite a cosmopolitan place. The original town was built in the 1600s and 1700s. It is a city of fabulous Spanish Colonial architecture and incredibly friendly citizens. Those are only a few of the reasons it is home to so many expats. The low cost of living is another, and that was definitely a factor in our decision to move there in March of 2014.

A majestic church, the Parroquia, watches over the city and directly before it sits the town square or Jardin. I had envisioned my future as sitting on a bench in the Jardin, watching the world go by and hoping I would remember my way home. If not, there are taxis everywhere, and I could keep my address in my pocket.

Thank God, my experience in San Miguel has been

nothing like I had imagined it. I had given myself a death sentence based on both my diagnosis and, the fact that, like most people, had no idea there existed the possibility of recovery.

I am in a very different space now than I was back then. I continue to take medication, though I am no longer sure that I need it, and I am following an exciting, recently developed treatment plan, the ReCODE (Reversing Cognitive Decline) Protocol, that for the first time in history is succeeding in reversing the symptoms of dementia in thousands of people.

Since I have made major changes to my lifestyle and the way I treat my body, changes that are integral to the ReCODE Protocol, the progression of my illness, mentally and physically, has been held at bay and, in multiple ways, improved dramatically. Most people today have no idea that I have or ever had a problem with cognition. Until now it has been believed impossible even to delay the progress of the disease, let alone recover from it.

I know that since I first heard of the protocol, and began to try and follow it, I have felt better physically and mentally than I have in many, many years. I no longer live with the certainty that I will soon die. I no longer dread social situations, and I am no longer making stupid mistakes on a daily basis. There is an entire later chapter that explains this protocol in depth. I also know for a fact that I now have something I haven't had in many years. That thing is HOPE.

My situation has changed dramatically for the better as a result of following the Protocol. There is no reason why your situation cannot improve as well. In the chapters that follow you are going to find information that can lift your spirits and head you in the direction of a life worth living. Until very recently it was thought that early diagnosis could not slow the progression of most types of dementia. That thinking is rapidly changing you, and are going to be introduced to the team of scientists responsible for that.

The ReCODE Protocol has been in existence for over five years now and is still relatively unknown. I am not following it perfectly, but within months of seriously implementing the changes in diet and lifestyle recommended, I experienced major improvement. After a few false starts, I have been practicing the program in earnest for about a year and a half. My situation should have deteriorated over that time frame, but instead, I continue to get better. It is too soon to know how long it will continue to work, but I have met people for whom it has continued to work for going on five years. Every day that I wake up feeling good and feeling hopeful, is to me a godsend. I had given up hope of ever having those types of days ever again, yet they continue to come, day after day.

In the following chapters, I will tell you more about my recovery and give you an overview of what I have learned about dementia and Alzheimer's. There will be helpful information for the twenty-five million plus caregivers, and more on the ReCODE Protocol. It is my hope that, if nothing else, I will make it clear that problems with memory do not always mean dementia, and that whatever your problem turns out to be, it may very well be REVERSIBLE.

MY INTRODUCTION TO THE BREDESEN PROTOCOL

It is May 2015, and I am in Novato, in northern California. It is the end of a long journey. Located in Marin County, 30 miles north of San Francisco, Novato is home to the Buck Institute for Research on Aging. It is also the location of one of Dr. Dale Bredesen's laboratories for the study of dementia. The Buck Institute was founded about seventeen years ago, and Dr. Bredesen was its first President and CEO. He has devoted decades to researching the causes of, and possible solutions for, memory problems associated with aging.

I first heard of Dr. Bredesen while having lunch in San Miguel de Allende, Mexico, with a group of expats who were all from 65 to 83 years of age. Someone mentioned that CNN had just done a story on a doctor who had succeeded in reversing symptoms of Alzheimer's Disease in nine out of ten patients. At that time, the doctor's treatment plan, ReCODE (Reversing Cognitive Decline), was being called the MEND Protocol."

Of course, I was interested, but I was also very skeptical. It seems like there is a story of another major breakthrough in Alzheimer's research every week, and most end up being just a headline to grab your attention, followed by nothing of real substance. Despite the fact that every single person at the table was experiencing at least some signs of memory loss, no one got very excited.

A few weeks later, I heard about it again and started looking into it. What I found out was nothing short of astounding, and since it was being presented by a joint team of researchers from both UCLA and The Buck Institute, it was credible.

In a small study that followed ten subjects for two and a half years, all of whom were exhibiting significant symptoms of dementia, a 36-point protocol based primarily on changes in lifestyle and nutrition had succeeded in reversing every symptom of Alzheimer's in all but one of the subjects. It is important to note that this study is now in its fifth year and all participants are still doing fine. In the last two years, Dr. Bredesen has continued his research, acquiring new information and incorporating that into what is now referred to as the ReCODE Protocol.

At the time I was learning about the doctor's major breakthrough, I had all but abandoned the idea of completing this book. While the existing manuscript, then titled *Descent into Dementia*, did offer a wealth of information on dementia, as well as many suggestions on how to cope with it, it also presented the story of an illness whose end was always the same: a long, painful decline, culminating in death. While it may have been helpful, it was also depressing. I was at a standstill with the book, and my own cognition had gotten to the point where I could no longer write coherently. For all practical purposes, the project was as dead as I expected to be in a few years.

Dr. Bredesen's research had provided the missing link, both for the book and also for my personal struggle with dementia. That link was A SOLUTION, something I had believed did not exist.

Although the original study included only ten subjects, less than three years later there were well over four hundred people following the ReCODE Protocol and experiencing the same success. That number is increasing every day as more people are learning about Dr. Bredesen's work. What follows is the introduction, three case studies, patients' stories, and the closing summary from the first report I read by Dr. Bredesen, "Reversal of Cognitive Decline: A Novel Therapeutic Program", published in Aging in September 2014. These will give you some insight into his approach.

Footnotes, acknowledgments, and references have been removed from the text of the report for ease of reading. These details are available at www.aging-us.com/article/100690/text. As this is a scientific document, it is rife with medical and scientific terms and I admit to not understanding all them. As the following are necessary to understand the treatment protocol, I have translated them for you, in the order in which they appear.

- po: by mouth
- qhs: every night
- bid: twice a day

INTRODUCTION

Magnitude of the problem

Cognitive decline is a major concern of the aging population, and Alzheimer's disease is the major cause of age-related cognitive decline, with approximately

5.4 million American patients and 30 million affected globally. In the absence of effective prevention and treatment, the prospects for the future are of great concern, with 13 million Americans and 160 million globally projected for 2050, leading to potential bankruptcy of the Medicare system. Unlike several other chronic illnesses, Alzheimer's disease prevalence is on the rise, which makes the need to develop effective prevention and treatment increasingly pressing. Recent estimates suggest that AD has become the third leading cause of death in the United States, behind cardiovascular disease and cancer. Furthermore, it has been pointed out recently that women are at the epicenter of the Alzheimer's epidemic, with 65% of patients and 60% of caregivers being women. Indeed, a woman's chance of developing AD is now greater than her chance of developing breast cancer.

CASE STUDIES

Patient one: history

A 67-year-old woman presented with two years of progressive memory loss. She held a demanding job that involved preparing analytical reports and traveling widely, but found herself no longer able to analyze data or prepare the reports, and therefore was forced to consider quitting her job. She noted that when she would read, by the time she reached the bottom of a page she would have to start at the top once again, since she was unable to remember the material she had just read. She was no longer able to remember numbers, and had to write down even 4- digit numbers to remember them. She also began to have trouble navigating on the road: even on familiar roads, she would become lost trying to figure out where to enter or exit the road. She also noticed that she would mix up the names of her pets, and forget where the light switches were in her home of years.

Her mother had developed similar progressive cognitive decline beginning in her early 60s, had become severely demented, entered a nursing home, and died at approximately 80 years of age.

When the patient consulted her physician about her problems, she was told that she had the same problem her mother had had, and that there was nothing he could do about it. He wrote "memory problems" in her chart, and therefore the patient was turned down in her application for long-term care.

After being informed that she had the same problem as her mother had had, she recalled the many years of her mother's decline in a nursing home. Knowing that there was still no effective treatment and subsequently losing the ability to purchase long-term care, she decided to commit suicide. She called a friend to commiserate, who suggested that she get on a plane and visit, and then referred her for evaluation.

She began System 1.0, and was able to adhere to some but not all of the protocol components. Nonetheless, after three months she noted that all of her symptoms had abated: she was able to navigate without problems, remember telephone numbers without difficulty, prepare reports and do all of her work without difficulty, read and retain information, and, overall, she became asymptomatic. She noted that her memory was now better than it had been in many years. On one occasion, she developed an acute viral illness, discontinued the program, and noticed a decline, which reversed when she reinstated the program. Two and one-half years later, now age 70, she remains asymptomatic and continues to work full-time.

Patient one: therapeutic program

As noted above, and following an extended discussion of the components of the therapeutic program, the patient began on some but not all of the system: (1) she eliminated all simple carbohydrates, leading to a weight loss of 20 pounds; (2) she eliminated gluten and processed food from her diet, and increased vegetables, fruits, and non-farmed fish; (3) in order to reduce stress, she began yoga, and ultimately became a yoga instructor; (4) as a second measure to reduce the stress of her job, she began to meditate for 20 minutes twice per day; (5) she took melatonin 0.5mg po qhs; (6) she increased her sleep from 4-5 hours per night to 7-8 hours per night; (7) she took methylcobalamin 1mg each day; (8) she took vitamin D3 2000IU each day; (9) she took fish oil 2000mg each day; (10) she took CoQ10 200mg each day; (11) she optimized her oral hygiene using an electric flosser and electric toothbrush; (12) following discussion with her primary care provider, she reinstated HRT (hormone replacement therapy) that had been discontinued following the WHI report in 2002; (13) she fasted for a minimum of 12 hours between dinner and breakfast, and for a minimum of three hours between dinner and bedtime; (14) she exercised for a minimum of 30 minutes, 4-6 days per week.

Patient two: history

A 69-year-old entrepreneur and professional man presented with 11 years of slowly progressive memory loss, which had accelerated over the past one or two years. In 2002, at the age of 58, he had been unable to recall the combination of the lock on his locker, and he felt that this was out of the ordinary for him. In 2003, he had FDG-PET (fluoro-deoxyglucose positron emission tomography), which was read as showing a pattern typical for early Alzheimer's disease, with reduced glucose utilization in the parietotemporal cortices bilaterally and left > right temporal lobes, but preserved utilization in the frontal lobes, occipital cortices, and basal ganglia. In 2003, 2007, and 2013, he had quantitative neuropsychological testing, which showed a reduction in CVLT (California Verbal Learning Test) from 84%ile to 1%ile, a Stroop color test at 16%ile, and auditory delayed memory at 13%ile. In 2013, he was found to be heterozygous for ApoE4 (3/4). He noted that he had progressive difficulty recognizing the faces at work (prosopagnosia), and had to have his assistants prompt him with the daily schedule. He also recalled an event during which he was several chapters into a book before he finally realized that it was a book he had read previously. In addition, he lost an ability he had had for most of his life: the ability to add columns of numbers rapidly in his head.

He had a homocysteine of 18 µmol/l, CRP <0.5mg/l, 25-OH cholecalciferol 28ng/ml, hemoglobin A1c 5.4%, serum zinc 78mcg/dl, serum copper 120mcg/dl, ceru-loplasmin 25mg/dl, pregnenolone 6ng/dl, testosterone 610ng/dl, albumin:globulin ratio of 1.3, cholesterol 165mg/dl (on Lipitor), HDL 92, LDL 64, triglyceride 47, AM cortisol 14mcg/dl, free T3 3.02pg/ml, free T4 1.27ng/l, TSH 0.58mIU/l, and BMI 24.9.

He began on the therapeutic program, and after six months, his wife, co-workers, and he all noted improvement. He lost 10 pounds. He was able to recognize faces at work unlike before, was able to remember his daily schedule, and was able to function at work without difficulty. He was also noted to be quicker with his responses. His life-long ability to add columns of numbers rapidly in his head, which he had lost during his progressive cognitive decline, returned. His wife pointed out that, although he had clearly shown improvement, the more striking effect was that he had been accelerating in his decline over the prior year or two, and this had been completely halted.

Patient two: therapeutic program

The patient began on the following parts of the overall therapeutic system: (1) he fasted for a minimum of three hours between dinner and bedtime, and for a minimum of 12 hours between dinner and breakfast; (2) he eliminated simple carbohydrates and processed foods from his diet; (3) he increased consumption of vegetables and fruits, and limited consumption of fish to non-farmed, and meat to occasional grass-fed beef or organic chicken; (4) he took probiotics; (5) he took coconut oil i tsp bid; (6) he exercised strenuously, swimming 3-4 times per week, cycling twice per week, and running once per week; (7) he took melatonin 0.5mg po qhs, and tried to sleep as close to 8 hours per night as his schedule would allow: (8) he took herbs Bacopa, monniera 250mg, Ashwagandha 500mg, and turmeric 400mg each day; (9) he took methylcobalamin 1mg, methyltetrahydrofolate 0.8mg, and pyridoxine-5-phosphate 50mg each day; (10) he took citicoline 500mg po bid; (11) he took vitamin C 1g per day, vitamin D3 5000IU per day, vitamin E 400IU per day, CoQ10 200mg per day, Zn picolinate 50mg per day, and α-lipoic acid 100mg per day; (12) he took DHA (docosahexaenoic acid) 320mg and EPA (eicosapentaenoic acid) 180mg per day.

Patient three: history

A 55-year-old attorney suffered progressively severe memory loss for four years. She accidentally left the stove on when she left her home on multiple occasions, and then returned, horrified to see that she had left it on once again. She would forget meetings, and agree to multiple meetings at the same time. Because of an inability to remember anything after a delay, she would record conversations, and she carried an iPad on which she took copious notes (but then forgot the password to unlock her iPad). She had been trying to learn Spanish as part of her job, but was unable to remember virtually anything new. She was unable to perform her job, and she sat her children down to explain to them that they could no longer take advantage of her poor memory, that instead they must understand that her memory loss was a serious problem. Her children noted that she frequently became lost in mid-sentence, that she was slow with responses, and that she frequently asked if they had followed up on something she thought she had asked them to do, when in fact she had never asked them to do the tasks to which she referred.

Her homocysteine was 9.8µmol/l, CRP 0.16mg/l, 25- OH cholecalciferol 46ng/ml, hemoglobin A1c 5.3%, pregnenolone 84ng/dl, DHEA 169ng/dl, estradiol 275pg/ml, progesterone 0.4ng/ml, insulin 2.7µIU/ml, AM cortisol 16.3mcg/dl, free T3 3.02pg/ml, free T4 1.32ng/l, and TSH 2.04mIU/l.

After five months on the therapeutic program, she noted that she no longer needed her iPad for notes, and no longer needed to record conversations. She was able to work once again, was able to learn Spanish, and began to learn a new legal specialty. Her children noted that she no longer became lost in mid- sentence, no longer thought she had asked them to do something that she had not asked, and answered their questions with normal rapidity and memory.

Patient three: therapeutic program

She began on the following parts of the therapeutic system: (1) she fasted for a minimum of three hours between dinner and bedtime, and for a minimum of 12 hours between dinner and breakfast; (2) she eliminated simple carbohydrates and processed foods from her diet; (3) she increased consumption of vegetables and fruits, limited consumption of fish to non-farmed, and did not eat meat; (4) she exercised 4- 5 times per week; (5) she took melatonin 0.5mg po qhs, and tried to sleep as close to 8 hours per night as her schedule would allow; (6) she tried to reduce stress in her life with meditation and relaxation; (7) she took methylcobalamin 1mg 4x/wk and pyridoxine-5- phosphate 20mg each day; (8) she took citicoline 200mg each day; (9) she took vitamin D3 2000IU per day and CoQ10200mg per day; (10) she took DHA 700mg and EPA 500mg bid; (11) her primary care provider prescribed bioidentical estradiol with estriol (BIEST), and progesterone; (12) her primary care provider worked with her to reduce her bupropion from 150mg per day to 150mg 3x/wk.

In Summary

A novel, comprehensive, and personalized therapeutic system is described that is based on the underlying pathogenesis of Alzheimer's disease. The basic tenets for the development of this system are also described.

Of the first 10 patients who utilized this program, including patients with memory loss associated with Alzheimer's disease (AD), amnestic mild cognitive impairment (aMCI), or subjective cognitive impairment (SCI), nine showed subjective or objective improvement.

One potentially important outcome is that all six of the patients whose cognitive decline had a major impact on job performance were able to return to work or continue working without difficulty.

These anecdotal results suggest the need for a controlled clinical trial of the therapeutic program.

Not long after I read this study, I started trying to implement the ReCODE Protocol on my own. Although the treatment plan for each individual is based on a host of information specific to that person, there was a lot of it I could begin right away. These were strategies that had been followed by everyone in the test group. My original efforts were in a way half-hearted. I was still not fully convinced it would work. I had been convinced for so long that I was dying it was difficult to make the switch in my thinking.

I began to experience a few changes in myself within a relatively short period of time. My physical health seemed to be improving and my spirits began to rise. I knew I had to contact this doctor, both for the book and for my own recovery.

When you accomplish something as extraordinary as reversing the symptoms of Alzheimer's, a disease forever thought to be both untreatable and fatal, you attract a lot of attention. Suddenly, Dr. Bredesen was swamped with invitations from all over the world to present his findings. It was no easy task to make contact with this man.

It started with an email. It took a while, but he responded. Not with the reply I had hoped for, but he responded. It took about two months of communicating with his assistant, Roweena Abulancia, to be able to speak with him on the telephone. But at 2 o'clock on a Friday afternoon in April of 2015, I found myself speaking to the man who was making history in the world of Alzheimer's studies.

I was anticipating a brief call of maybe five minutes during which I would plead for a face-to-face interview.

After being on Larry King Live, CNN, and featured in the New York Times, I assumed Dr. Bredesen would have very little time for me, an unknown writer in Mexico. Asking him for a half-hour interview seemed like a pretty long shot. I thought there was a good chance he would be somewhat arrogant and dismiss my request out of hand. Roweena, when she put him on the phone, suggested I be as concise as possible as I would probably only have a few minutes to speak to him.

Imagine my elation when I discovered he was anything but arrogant. Rather, the Doctor proved to be a very kind and friendly man who seemed more interested in talking about my own experience with dementia than he was in talking about himself. We spoke for almost half an hour. He seemed to be listening to me more attentively than any of my own doctors ever had.

I finally got the conversation back to him. Not only did he consent to an interview, but he also invited me to attend an event at the Buck Institute where he was going to present his findings to a group of about 150 people, some of whom had dementia and were already following his protocol with amazing results. Making the trip at the time seemed like a big expense but, I can tell you that beyond a shadow of a doubt, it was the best money I ever spent in my entire life.

The first speaker was a woman, known as Julie Gee, who had experienced every single symptom of dementia that I had. Like me, she had been forced to drop out of the workplace, no longer able to practice a profession she had been in for years. She also had experienced problems with driving, finding herself getting lost while being in an area she had been living for a very long time. I had never actually gotten lost, but I was frequently finding myself heading in the wrong direction or forgetting where it was I was going to.

On her own, with no help from anyone, she had conducted research and had begun to adopt many of the lifestyle changes she would later learn were part of Dr. Bredesen's protocol. She had added many elements of his plan to her own regime, and the recovery she was experiencing was not only astounding, it was real, right there in front of me. As I listened and observed, I could detect absolutely no sign of any kind of cognitive impairment. She presented herself with a confidence that I had not been capable of for several years.

Later in the day I approached Julie and introduced myself. We agreed to get in contact with one another at a later date. After a number of phone conversations, I learned that she spends enormous amounts of her time helping others to recover from dementia. The website www.apoe4.info has been a clearinghouse for information on Alzheimer's for several years. She was instrumental in the creation of that resource.

Originally www.apoe4.info was a chat room for people with the gene ApoE4 to exchange information on how they were dealing with cognitive decline. Today it is an invaluable source offering useful information in almost daily updates. If anything, anywhere is showing success in testing Alzheimer's it will soon appear on the site.

An article from CNN Health, December 8, 2014, tells some of Julie's story. Sections of this article, which do not specifically refer to her have been removed. The entire article can be
found at
http://edition.cnn.com/2014/12/08/health/alzheimers-reversal/index.html

> *The woman at the department store bounded toward Julie Gee.*
>
> *"Julie! Hi! How have you been?" she asked. Gee, 49, stared blankly at her. A few uncomfortable seconds passed.*
>
> *"I have no idea who this woman is," Gee* thought. She felt herself slipping into a sort of cognitive abyss.*
>
> *"Remember, our sons went to school together?" the woman said. "We did playground duty together?" Gee's mind was dark. She began to panic.*
>
> *"I tried to act like I sort of knew who she was, became visibly upset and just left the store," she said, recalling the scenario years later. "It was horrible, just terrifying."*
>
> *That painful interaction was the first sign of Gee's early stage Alzheimer's disease, which genetic tests later confirmed.*

Her memory lapses mounted: Gee would find herself, for a few seconds at a time, forgetting where she was while driving familiar roads. She would walk away from conversations with her husband mid- sentence. She would be reading and unable to relate, moments later, even a shred of what she had just read.

The idea of a long, painful descent into Alzheimer's was too much to bear. Gee's initial fear after her diagnosis metastasized to hopelessness.

"I seriously considered suicide," she said.

Not long after her memory problems began, Gee found out she carries two copies of the APOE-4 allele. Simply put, this gene hampers her brain's ability to heal itself, dramatically increasing her risk for developing Alzheimer's disease.

It was the final straw.

Gee threw herself into reading studies, gathering information and implementing any lifestyle change that might slow down her disease. Later, she said, she sought help from a well-known neurologist, Dr. David Perlmutter, who helped her to refine those changes.

As it turns out, Perlmutter's advice in many ways mirrored Bredesen's program.

Gee began by adding fish oil and other supplements to her daily regimen. In several studies, people who took the supplements performed better on memory tests and had bigger brains. She also started meditating twice daily and sleeping seven to eight hours each night; adequate sleep and exercise improve blood flow to the brain and instigate neuron generation.

Hormone replacement therapy is indicated for women who have a hormonal imbalance that may be affecting brain function, so Gee started that too.

She fasts for more than 12 hours between dinner and the next day's breakfast, making sure there are at least three hours between dinner and bedtime. The idea behind fasting, said Bredesen, is that with the break the body begins a process called autophagy, which can help destroy amyloid-beta, a problematic protein that builds up in the brains of Alzheimer's patients.

Gee has also cut out processed foods from her diet, including sugar, grains and other starches, since they can stir up inflammation in the brain. Her rule of thumb: "I don't buy any packaged, boxed or canned food."

A typical dinner for her includes mostly raw organic vegetables drizzled with extra virgin olive oil and wild caught fish. Occasionally she replaces the fish with grass-fed lean meats. She has integrated more fermented foods into her diet — research is beginning to correlate gut health with brain health.

"Piece by piece I was going down the protocol,"

> *she said. "My mental acuity improved the more (elements of the program) I began doing."*
>
> *The overhaul Gee and others did would be dizzying for most people, but Gee said it had the converse effect of simplifying her life. She said cutting out so much processed and other inflammatory foods is freeing.*
>
> *Within a few months of beginning the protocol she said she experienced a dramatic cognitive turnaround. Gee had been testing in the 30th percentile on an online brain training website before the program. Months afterward, she was scoring above the 90th percentile.*
>
> *"Before this protocol, the notion was you were going to die with this disease," said Gee, who started a website to provide support and hope for others in the same genetic situation. "There was a lack of specificity about what to do. Now we have this prevention protocol."*

The next speaker was the doctor himself. The title of the day's event was THE DAWN OF THE AGE OF REVERSIBLE ALZHEIMER'S. Later in the afternoon, I had the opportunity to spend time with him alone. He explained the science behind his protocol in as simple terms as possible. At that time the protocol, then being called the MEND Protocol, had been in existence for over four years. He has learned much in the following years and made adjustments and additions to his program as new information emerged. It was to be another two years before the final protocol, now called ReCODE (Reversing Cognitive Decline) was introduced to the world in his book *The End of Alzheimer's*.

Dr. Bredesen told me that while most of the scientific community have been trying to find a single cause for the disease of Alzheimer's, his research and that of others have isolated thirty-six separate culprits that are linked to cognitive impairment in study after study. He said that trying to treat the illness based on any one single cause was like patching one hole in a roof that, in fact, had thirty-six holes.

While you may not have the opportunity to speak with him personally, his recently published book lays out the entire science behind the protocol as well as exactly what you need to do to implement it. It is very easy to read and, in my opinion, life-saving information. The first chapter, "How to Give Yourself Alzheimer's" describes in detail the life I was living before learning of the path to recovery that I follow today.

Dr. Bredesen's treatment plan involves individual testing to determine which of the possible thirty-six potential factors are at play. Not every person will have all, or even most, of the possible problems in evidence. Once the potential sources of the illness are identified, they can then be targeted. The treatment is not complicated, but it is for some quite difficult because it involves making changes to ways of living and eating that some people are not willing to do.

Much has changed since I met Dr. Bredesen over two years ago from the date of this writing. He sees the ReCODE Protocol as not just a cure for Alzheimer's, but a design for living that will eliminate the possibility of getting the disease in the first place. He believes everyone can benefit from practicing the protocol before any signs of cognitive impairment surface.

Research has discovered a direct link between the possibility of getting Alzheimer's and the presence of certain genes, particularly the gene ApoE4. Persons with this gene have significantly greater odds of acquiring the disease. The doctor believes anyone with this gene should start practicing the ReCODE plan immediately.

In the desire to make ReCODE available to as many people as possible, he founded a company called AHNP: Precision Health. For the last year and a half, they have been training doctors all over the country to be able to treat patients using the protocol.

AHNP is now offering immersion programs which, as the name suggests, will, over several days, teach you everything you need to know to get started practicing the protocol in your own life. As part of the immersion program, you will receive the individualized testing necessary to create your treatment plan and you will be assigned a doctor to monitor your case for one year. A nutritionist will assist you in formulating a diet plan, and you will be given a one-year supply of nutritional supplements needed to counter any deficiencies detected, as well as those suggested as a matter of course. You will learn of the link between stress and Alzheimer's and be offered suggestions on how to reduce it. There will be instruction on meditation and opportunities to practice. If you are interested in attending one of these immersion programs visit their website at www.ahnphealth.com.

As you can see from the report on the original study, a major component of the ReCODE Protocol concerns diet, which is not to be confused with dieting. Dr. Bredesen is convinced that healthy eating is necessary for a healthy mind, and the protocol involves what for many will be a radical change in eating habits. The hardest part for me was eliminating refined sugar, processed foods, and gluten, all of which have been directly linked to cognitive impairment. I never realized how fond I was of junk food before I tried to eliminate it, and my inability to do so right away hindered my process of recovery for many months.

My wife has been instrumental in helping me adopt the changes to diet that are a critical component of this protocol. I asked her today how she felt about facilitating these changes, and the recovery she has seen in how I think and act. Her exact reply was, "Fantastic. I wish I was doing more, but it has been wonderful." There were several years when she had been living with nothing but fear and despair. To hear that she felt fantastic was music to my ears.

The following chapter will show you how I finally came to follow all of the protocol to the best of my ability and how I became convinced that the treatment could and, in fact, did restore my cognitive function and return me to a life worth living.

HOW I AM RECOVERING FROM ALZHEIMER'S

The process of learning about and implementing the ReCODE (Reversing Cognitive Decline) Protocol into my life has not been a straight line. After reading the report that I reprinted in the preceding chapter, it was over a year before I became completely convinced that it was working and totally committed myself to trying my absolute best to practice it in my life on a daily basis. It was over another year after that that I read Dr. Bredesen's *The End of Alzheimer's* and gained a much clearer understanding of what I should be doing.

By the time I went to Novato, met Dr. Bredesen, and saw firsthand the results people were getting from the protocol, I had already been doing some of the things suggested, but not all. I was having a great deal of trouble coming to terms with not eating refined sugar or products containing gluten, particularly bread and pasta.

I was taking some of the supplements suggested, and I was beginning to meditate and exercise more regularly. I had already done much to eliminate the stress in my life by exiting the workforce and moving to Mexico, and I was getting the suggested number of hours of sleep every night. It was the change in eating habits that was presenting the biggest challenge.

The ReCODE Protocol also calls for fasting 12 hours between dinner and breakfast. This proved for me to be very difficult. I have been a midnight snacker all my life, and to this day, although I am much improved, I have not broken the habit altogether.

It is important to remember that to practice the protocol optimally it is necessary to be thoroughly tested to determine which of the 36 potential factors leading to Alzheimer's are at play. The average person experiencing cognitive decline of the Alzheimer's type has 10 to 25 things that need to be dealt with, and you can only know what many of them are through testing.

Living in Mexico, much of this testing was either not available or not within my means to pay for. In the United States, most insurance companies will pay for the great majority of the tests, if not all. I had some blood work done that showed some nutritional deficiencies, which I was able to address immediately. After that, I simply began doing almost all of the things the three patients in the case histories had done. I did not immediately switch to eating all organic foods, but I did make multiple changes in my diet.

I eliminated almost all refined sugar from my diet. I was surprised to discover how pervasive the presence of sugar was in the things I had been eating. I had never suspected that there was sugar in things like condiments and salad dressing. Every time I discovered I was eating something with sugar hidden away among the ingredients, I eliminated it. I also eliminated all gluten. We struggled to find gluten-free bread that tasted like bread and had very little luck, so I simply stopped eating breads and rolls. I do allow myself a roll at Thanksgiving and Christmas dinner. We did eventually find gluten-free pasta that is delicious.

For the first time in my life, I began to have fresh salads every day. To my surprise, I learned to enjoy them. There is very little use of fertilizers in the area of Mexico in which I live, so it is easy to find organic vegetables. In addition to vegetables, I introduced fish to my diet. The plan suggests eating wild, not farm grown, red fish. I now eat salmon for dinner three times a week. I also eat red snapper somewhat frequently. I had been eating tuna, but Dr. Bredesen suggests that since that type of fish is likely to contain high levels of mercury it should be avoided or eaten in moderation. That is one of the many things I learned from reading his book. What I also learned from the book was that the tropical fruits in the smoothies I had been starting many days with were not beneficial for me. I am now using berries and protein powder.

After my time with the doctor, I began taking every supplement that had been mentioned in the original study. And I began seeing major improvement very quickly. I had met Dr. Bredesen in May, and by October I was feeling very much like my old self, after a mere five and a half months of closely following the plan as I understood it at that time. My memory was still not at 100 percent, but it was greatly improved.

Then something happened. I was talking with a group of people about gaining and losing weight, and a woman asked me exactly how much I weighed. At that point, I had lost about 45 pounds, 15 of which I had lost prior to moving to Mexico and learning of the protocol. One of the rare side effects of Aricept is a loss of appetite, and I had by then been taking the drug for around three years.

When I told her my weight, she said, "No man should weigh that little." I was embarrassed and felt diminished. I told myself the next day that I would gain some weight quickly.

I was planning to go to the border a few days later, and I was traveling alone. That was significant because when my thinking was at its worst, I was very reluctant to travel anywhere without a companion. The last time I had done so, I found myself on the wrong plane at one point and got lost in a terminal at another. I also managed to leave my favorite hat on one of the planes. That I could now comfortably travel solo was for me more proof that I was getting better.

I spent three and a half days at the border, and while there I binged continuously on things like ice cream, licorice, peanut butter, and cinnamon rolls. I even went to a McDonalds one day. And yes, I gained weight. About five pounds.

I had assumed that when I got back to San Miguel, I would just resume my good eating habits. That did not happen. Although I was no longer eating everything in sight, I did continue to eat some refined sugar products, and I also started to forget to take my supplements on schedule. And, for some reason, I had let up on my exercise program, not altogether but I was not exercising as rigorously as before.

About a week after I returned from the border, perhaps a little longer, I am not sure, my cognitive abilities took a severe turn for the worse. It did not happen immediately, it deteriorated a day at a time. Two or possibly three weeks after being back home I could no longer hold a thought for the time it took to cross a room. My memory had returned to almost the same condition it was in before I had ever heard of Dr. Bredesen and his life-saving work. It was very scary.

Once I became aware of how bad things had become, I recommitted myself to practicing the protocol and returned to it convinced that I could not take vacations from it. I needed to devote myself to this new way of living or risk a relapse.

My cognition did not improve immediately. It was several months before I started to feel like I had before dropping my regimen. There were a few times when I thought I would never regain the improvements I had originally experienced.

Talking on the phone one evening with Thom Mount,

I was very relieved to hear that my experience was not unique. Many of the participants in the original study, as well as many who have begun following the ReCODE Protocol in the last two years, had experienced the same thing and their cognition did return. That conversation gave me the encouragement I needed to press on. I am very grateful to Mr. Mount for sharing that information.

One last word about food. The plan calls for the elimination of processed food. Dr. Bredesen's book defines processed food as anything that lists the ingredients. While I have removed much of the processed food from my diet, I would be lying if I said I had eliminated all. It is one of the parts of the protocol that I am working to improve on. My entire experience with this new way of living has been a process of continually improving, adding new aspects of the plan as I become aware of them, and working to improve on the things I am doing. Having recently read *The End of Alzheimer's*, I intend to have additional testing done this week and tweak my food plan and supplement intake accordingly.

The protocol recommends vigorous aerobic exercise several times per week for 30 to 45 minutes. Some people exercise as many as six days per week, some fewer. In the beginning, I was walking briskly about two miles every day. I have now increased that to a goal of 10,000 steps daily, which I keep track of on my iPhone. Many phones have this feature and there are apps available. I reach my goal about three times a week, the other days I manage about five to nine thousand steps.

With my stride, ten thousand steps are a little short of five miles. San Miguel is a very hilly town, so the walking is great aerobic exercise. I also work with a small set of weights a few times a week to gain muscle strength.

The part of my program that I enjoy the most is meditation. Even though I am semi-retired, I still manage to find ways to stress myself out sometimes. I try to meditate a minimum of five times weekly. I belong to two groups that practice together once a week and I practice at home almost every day. I simply sit quietly, focus on my breathing, and try to free my mind from all negative thoughts. I try to catch myself when I let any thoughts in, acknowledge them, and let them go. I find doing this for as little as five minutes is beneficial, but I strive for twenty. When I get away from the practice, I will start feeling differently after a week or so. I will find myself getting stressed out and I will regress.

I mentioned earlier that I do my best to get eight to nine hours of sleep nightly. I have never had very good sleep habits, and what now makes this possible for me is that I take melatonin before bed every night. While I do not always reach my goal, I am sleeping better than I ever have before. My wife says melatonin gives her strange dreams. Fortunately, that has not been my experience.

Please do not think that reading my book is a substitute for seeing a doctor and being introduced to the ReCODE Protocol by a trained professional. I have been extremely blessed to have experienced the recovery I have with very little supervision. I am certain that were I to live in the States and have access to treatment, I would be even healthier than I am. While I am certain that my cognition is infinitely better than it was four years ago, I do acknowledge that there is still room for improvement. I am confident that as I add aspects of the protocol that I learned about in *The End of Alzheimer's* it will improve even more.

There are a few other things I do as part of my personal plan of recovery on a daily basis. As suggested by the protocol, I practice optimal oral hygiene. This is important because any type of inflammation can have an effect on the brain's ability to keep producing healthy neurons. And, it is something everyone learned from their Moms to do.

I feel compelled to mention two more aspects of my personal program of recovery. One is that I have been blessed with a very strong faith for many, many years. From the day I first saw my diagnosis in print, I was convinced that no matter what happened I would be okay. I do not believe this higher power I choose to call God shields us from bad things happening. We see the truth of that every day. I do believe, however, that we are given what we need to survive these difficult experiences intact. First among these gifts is our fellow man, the people in our lives we can turn to for support when life seems overwhelming. I can think of no other reason that people survive tragedies every day and come out the other side able to go on. I was convinced from day one, that with the help of my family and friends I would be okay. I might become extremely ill and eventually die, but I would be okay during the process. I would not be alone.

Which brings me to my beautiful wife, Patricia. We met when we were very young, and our lives changed forever. We have had many wonderful times together, times of incredible joy. And like any couple that has been together for forty years, we have experienced real pain. At the age of thirty-two, my wife was stricken with a major illness and it became my job to take care of her basic needs for several years. It was a labor of love. It was 27 years later, decades after she had made a remarkable recovery, that I was diagnosed with pre-senile dementia. From that moment to this, she has been instrumental in my being able to follow the protocol. She spent hours searching out sources for healthy foods and experimenting with recipes to make them taste good. She has been the one to find affordable sources for the supplements I take, and she has been the one to make sure they are always in supply. And early on, it was Pat that reminded me to take them twice a day.

In the beginning, doing things like finding an electric toothbrush was too much for me to remember. But one showed up in my bathroom. Guess who bought it? While that assistance was invaluable in helping with the mechanics of following the protocol, it was the least of it.

From the very start, she reassured me on dozens of

occasions that I would be okay. Whenever I was having a particularly hard time and thinking that the protocol wasn't working, she would always assure me that it was, that I was just having a bad day. Our relationship is such that I never doubted for a second that she would stay with me to the end, whatever that looked like. She may have told me that, but it wasn't necessary.

I am certain that none of this has been easy for her. Our former life was one of little worry. She had never had to think about her future security. She hadn't worked in thirty years and didn't need to. She was a full-time Mom, and that was fine with her and me. Our situation changed radically in every way when I became ill. Our entire financial situation took a severe turn for the worse as I continued to deny my illness and make endless errors of judgment in the process.

This had to have been enormously stressful for her, but she maintained a positive attitude from then until now. I have no doubt in my mind that without her I would not have recovered.

So that is how I did it, and with the new information I gained in The End of Alzheimer's, I am adding to my program. Yours will not be the same as mine, but if you follow the instructions you are given, you are almost certain to experience similar results. Better in fact, because you will not be delaying the way I was.

Everyone who sees one of AHNP's doctors and receives the appropriate testing will end up following a slightly different program, specific to themselves. The program I have been following, while no doubt not the perfect plan for me, has been working. But I implore you to not just start doing the one I have presented. Though nothing in it will hurt you and all of what I have done will help, it is not the ReCODE Protocol if you don't get tested by a trained physician before you start.

What You Can Do Today?

Equally as important as what you can do today is what you should not do. DO NOT be overwhelmed by the seeming difficulty of the Protocol. Dr. Bredesen suggests that you do not have to do everything at once. Get started with whatever aspect of the plan you think you can do and add to it as you go along.

Another thing you should not do is to tell yourself you are not that bad, that you will try it when it gets worse. Your denial system is always going to be telling you it is not that bad until the point when it is very bad. The disease started long before you were aware of it and it is progressing continually if nothing is done to stop it. I had lunch yesterday with a friend who is both aware of my situation and having cognitive difficulties of his own. They are obvious to me. But he is, "not that bad," so he is changing nothing. Don't be like him

What you absolutely should do as soon as possible is obtain a copy of Dr. Bredesen's book *The End of Alzheimer's*. It is available on Amazon as well as is in most major bookstores. In it you will find absolutely everything you need to do to begin to recover. Dr. Bredesen is a very empathetic man. He understands that parts of his protocol are not easy at first. His book is designed to inform you rather than overwhelm you. He emphasizes at many points that probably no one is doing all of it, that in fact you probably do not need all of it.

Contact AHNP: Precision Health. You can find contact information on their website www.ahnphealth.com and get referred to one of their trained physicians near you. Attend an immersion program if possible. Start today. The sooner you begin addressing your problem the sooner it will begin to go away.

That is really all you need to do. That and follow the suggestions in the book. If you want to get started before you see a doctor, there are simple things you can do to begin. Start exercising. Try to reduce whatever stress is in your life. Start removing refined sugar from your diet and stop eating processed food. As I hope I made clear, I did not profoundly change my diet at first. It took months to get comfortable living without sweets and consuming more healthy foods.

Is it easy? No, it is not. But when you consider the choices are to either do it or die an ugly death from a horrible disease, it is not a difficult decision to make. At least it was not for me.

The good news is that today, over two and a half years since my meeting with Dr. Bredesen, I feel like my mind is functioning the best it has been in many years. I asked my wife recently if she still felt like she was living with someone with dementia and she said, without hesitation,

"No." I asked her that question because for the last few months there have been many days I no longer feel like a person that ever had dementia. I am certain my memory is not perfect, but I do not think it is worse than most of my friends in their sixties or older. In fact, I know it is better than a lot of them. I have to admit, I do have an occasional day when my memory seems worse than usual. I believe these are times when I may have let my guard down on what I am eating, or I have developed some unaddressed stress in my life. Those days give me a renewed commitment to following the protocol to the absolute best of my ability.

I also know that if I discontinue doing what I have been doing for the last two years I will lose all the progress I have gained. Mr. Mount told me recently that approximately 85 percent of the people who practice the ReCODE Protocol vigorously have the same positive result that I have experienced. They reverse the symptoms of dementia! To this day, many still believe that that is an impossibility. As a person who has been given my life back, I know that is simply antiquated thinking.

Those who do not recover are the people for whom the disease is so far progressed that they are unable to practice the program. They lack the awareness to stay focused on what they are doing. I know if I had not had my wife to help me with some of the things I mentioned earlier, I probably would not have experienced the success that I have.

I also know that if you have the desire to recover and the willingness to make some changes in your life, the ReCODE protocol can work for you as well. The only side effects that have been reported by any of the participants are weight loss, more energy, and an improved outlook on life. The weight loss I experienced was a result of medication I was taking more than the protocol. I have since managed to arrive at a comfortable and correct body mass.

Five years ago, I dreaded getting out of bed in the morning. I had no idea what blunder I would make, what inappropriate word would come out of my mouth, who I would offend by not recognizing them, which unfulfilled promise I would be reminded of, or even if I would survive the day without another car accident. I had given up all hope for my future, and I was worried sick about my wife's financial security, or lack of same. Thoughts of suicide were my constant companions.

Today I wake up eager to see what the world has to offer. I make new friends all the time and I am not afraid I will forget them by the afternoon. My wife recently told me she would like to visit the highlands in Scotland, home of her ancestors. Today I can once again make plans, and I believe it's possible we may actually do just that. My thirty-year-old son recently fell in love. I am thinking I may live long enough to meet my grandchildren. Life is good today, and I believe it will only get better.

I am convinced that it is only by the grace of God that

I overheard that first conversation about Dr. Bredesen. To this day I have yet to meet a person in Mexico, other than the few people who were present at that time, who has even heard his name. And I talk to people who are worried about their own or a loved one's cognition almost every week. I am not afraid to talk about my experience with anyone who has a desire to know more about Alzheimer's. Once again, if you are worried about cognitive decline in your own or anyone else's life, I implore you to read *The End of Alzheimer's*. Do not give up hope. A solution is at hand; you need only be willing to look for it.

TO THE CAREGIVERS

I recently reread this chapter for the first time in almost a year. It occurred to me that since the advent of the Bredesen Protocol, millions of people are going to be spared the need for much of what is written here. Hopefully, in the not too distant future, the possibility of recovering from Alzheimer's will be so well known that few people will reach the point of needing full-time care. In the meantime, however, there are millions of people who do, and so this chapter is dedicated to those who provide that care.

Several months ago, I had coffee with Don Cramer, author of the recently released book, Where is Whitney Now? Like me, it was Alzheimer's that brought him to San Miguel de Allende. Originally from San Diego, California, Don took care of his wife for ten years, as she progressed through the stages of Alzheimer's. They eventually reached a point in their journey where she needed more care than Don was capable of providing.

When Don began looking for a facility that would provide the level of care for his wife that he wished for, he soon discovered that in the United States such facilities are enormously expensive, and were out of his reach financially. Through a series of coincidences (which by the way he does not believe in), he learned about San Miguel and the fact that it was home to a world-class care facility, Cielito Lindo, for people suffering from dementia.

After just one visit to Cielito Lindo, Don was convinced that this was the place he had been looking for. In addition to a beautiful setting, the main attraction for Don was the level of care being provided for the residents. As Don says, "It's a special place where residents are considered family and loving care happens as a way of life." And, fortunately for the Cramers, it was within their means.

Very shortly after visiting San Miguel and touring the facility, Don realized two things. One, he could move to this magical town in the mountains of Mexico and be perfectly content. Americans and Canadians had been moving to San Miguel for decades. And two, he knew that Cielito Lindo was the best place for Whitney he would ever find. He would be able to visit her every day, and when he wasn't there, he could be content trusting her care to their dedicated, attentive staff.

I highly recommend his book to anyone who is taking care of a loved one with Alzheimer's. It is a very moving account of both the difficulties of caring for a loved one as they progress through the disease, as well as an inspirational portrayal of transforming a very difficult situation into a love story.

When I was speaking with Don, I felt a sense of guilt. Unlike Whitney, I had been fortunate enough to have been exposed to Dr. Bredesen's work, and I am in the process of recovering from what I once thought was an incurable disease. Many people, including most doctors, still believe that dementia is incurable. I could tell from our conversation that Don had searched high and low for help for his wife and had sadly encountered some charlatans along the way. Fortunately for me, both Dr. Bredesen and the facilities where he did his research, UCLA and The Buck Institute, are highly regarded and well respected. I sensed that Don had been led astray with false hopes so many times that he was very skeptical of my own story.

Taking care of a family member with dementia will probably be the most difficult task you will ever be called upon to perform. It is physically, emotionally and mentally challenging, and it becomes harder as the disease progresses. Dealing with a person afflicted with dementia requires all the patience, love, tolerance, understanding, and kindness you can muster. However, it may also provide you with opportunities to experience love from and express love for that person that you never imagined. It will definitely be challenging, but as Mr. Cramer's book makes clear, it can also be incredibly rewarding.

There are usually many years between the onset of dementia of the Alzheimer's type and the person's passing. You are entering a period when the amount of help you can muster for yourself will be directly linked to not only the quality of care you will be able to provide for your loved one but the quality of your own life as well. Hopefully, this chapter will make the search for that help easier.

The good news is that YOU ARE NOT ALONE. The Alzheimer's Association estimates that there are approximately 25 million people currently providing care for people with this disease, most of them family members. Other estimates are even higher. And this number only includes the caregivers who are not paid, those who labor for love.

Society has recognized the toll Alzheimer's has taken on those who are called upon to assume the role, and as a result, there are a number of both national and community-based programs and organizations dedicated to helping these caregivers.

Recent studies have shown that caregivers are prone not only to emotional difficulties but physical maladies as well. Therefore, not only is proper care necessary for the patient's well-being, the one giving that care needs to monitor their own health closely as well.

The financial future of the caregiver may also be at stake. A person that is cognitively impaired can do great harm to the family's finances, as I did, and not even realize it.

Based on my family's experience, and at the risk of sounding cold, it needs to be said that some of the most important work that will need to be done is limiting losses to the family's financial well-being. This can often be most critical in the earliest stages of the illness when the patient is still working. Poor choices and impulsive decisions can do great harm in this era when stocks can be bought and sold with the push of a button and money can be transferred from one account to another with great ease.

I was running a small business at the time my symptoms became problematic. It was a small business because I was no longer capable of running a large one. Although only six years earlier I had been the Executive Director of a large not for profit corporation, responsible for dozens of employees in two countries, I could no longer manage even a handful of employees. In fact, I could no longer even manage myself. I was losing large sums of money on a regular basis without even being aware of it.

During this period, I was working in the construction industry, and the losses were directly accountable to the fact that not only was I underestimating the projects I was doing, I was also failing to manage their proper execution. I was borrowing money from my retirement account on a regular basis and I would either forget to repay these loans to myself or not remember having made them, thus giving the business the appearance of at least breaking even. I think in my desire to keep my problems hidden from others, I was also somehow hiding them from myself.

All this time, my wife would have been, and continues to be, quite capable of helping me see, and perhaps mitigate, the damage being done - if I had let her. Truth be known, eventually, she tried to do that more than once, and I only became defensive. For the first couple of years I was losing money, she had no idea that I might have some form of cognitive impairment, and she did not realize the extent of the losses. She spent very little time thinking about things financial. She was accustomed to knowing we were very comfortable in that regard. I was unaware of them myself.

Eventually, it became clear to her that I was making a lot of poor decisions, that I needed help running my business and that I was putting our future at risk. Partially because I was too proud, and in part, because I still believed I could figure out what was happening and rectify the problem on my own, I was not open to accepting that help. I was in total denial that anything was wrong with my thinking.

By the time she was completely aware of our situation, it was almost too late. I had pretty much depleted a lifetime of savings and investments. Our only remaining asset was our one home in the Caribbean, which fortunately for us we had owned for decades. I cannot overemphasize the importance of helping your loved one recognize his problem when he is in denial of it. Follow your gut; it will know when something is seriously wrong.

People with cognitive impairment forget things constantly, including that they have a problem. They are capable of looking in disbelief at a savings or brokerage account statement one day and then not think about it again for weeks on end. The next time they look, things have gotten worse. The process of being shocked, and then forgetting again, occurs repeatedly.

That may not happen to everyone who is cognitively impaired, but it happened to me. In my arrogance, every time I became aware of the situation, I would somehow convince myself I could turn our financial problems around, and things would be okay again, one day soon. That day never came. And in my illness, I kept forgetting.

It is imperative that, from the moment you first suspect that something is amiss, you begin paying close attention to all things related to finance. Bank balances need to be monitored and a close eye kept on the checkbook.

If your loved one has always been quite capable in the past, do not assume he still is. When will you know it’s time to start paying more attention? There will be warning signs. Keys or wallets may seem to be constantly misplaced. Appointments and commitments will be forgotten or overlooked. There will begin to be events happening that just don't seem to go as planned. And your loved one may become defensive about conversations related to business or finances in general.

One of the ingredients in any healthy relationship is communication. Talk to your loved one. Share with him what you have been noticing. Try and determine if he is aware of them as well. Perhaps refer to something you have forgotten yourself recently, see if he identifies. If there is a business involved, get a look at the books, more than one look. Try to remember this is going to be a very sensitive issue for the one you love. Admitting to having problems with your brain is a difficult, painful task that most people do not want to do, even to themselves.

What often happens when problems begin to surface is the phenomenon of denial. No one, neither the persons afflicted nor the people who love them, wants to admit there could be something seriously wrong. And so, they rationalize and minimize the things that are occurring. The tendency is to attribute the difficulties to stress, overwork or just growing older: anything but dementia.

DO NOT MINIMIZE OR RATIONALIZE SIGNS OF IMPAIRMENT. At some point, it will be necessary to remove your loved one's access to banking activities altogether, but it is never too early to start keeping a close eye on things.

A certain amount of forgetfulness is a natural part of the aging process. Almost everyone starts to have occasional lapses in memory as they grow older. This is not a cause for concern. However, when it starts happening almost every day, or tasks that once were accomplished with ease are becoming problematic, it is time to investigate.

If the afflicted person has historically been the one responsible for the preparation and payment of income taxes, it is time to get involved. Not only is difficulty with math part and parcel of the disease, it is also possible this task is being forgotten altogether or being ignored due to the difficulty of dealing with it. People with dementia tend to avoid those things that confront them with their own inadequacies. Tax preparation, or any task that requires clear thinking, is likely to be postponed and perhaps forgotten altogether. You do not want to allow problems to develop in this area when so many other things are beginning to go awry.

If you have not used a tax consultant in the past, it may be time to do so now. If you do have someone that helps with the taxes, contact them and make sure everything is in order.

Caring for a person with Alzheimer's requires almost constant awareness. It becomes increasingly important to monitor all areas of responsibility that have previously been theirs. It will fall on the caregiver to ensure that all the bills are being paid. If you have a mortgage, make certain payments are being made. You need to protect not only your assets but your credit rating as well.

You may also want to start monitoring your loved one's driving skills. It is not uncommon for people with cognitive impairment to have difficulties paying attention at the wheel or responding rapidly to conditions they encounter.

I had several little fender benders during the early

stages of my difficulties. That was one of the reasons we moved to a small town. I would be able to walk wherever I needed to go, and hopefully not get lost if my condition worsened. That was the thinking at the time, but my condition has improved rather than deteriorated. I am happy to report that a few months ago we bought a car and I am now driving on a regular basis and feeling comfortable doing so. That is just one of dozens of ways in which my life has dramatically changed since implementing the ReCODE Protocol.

At some point in the progression of the disease, it will become obvious that the driver is a safety hazard to herself and others. This will be a very difficult period for her. The ability to go anywhere when you want to is one of the basic rights of adulthood. It is a symbol of our independence. For years the automobile has been a cornerstone of the American Dream. It is no surprise that there will be great reluctance to forfeiting that right.

You are likely to encounter resistance when you try and broach this subject. It is often a good idea to let the family doctor relay this information for you. A doctor's opinion is sometimes easier to accept than that of a family member. In whatever way this is done, you owe it to both the one you are caring for, as well as society in general, to make sure the keys get put away at the appropriate time.

The farther the dementia advances, the more difficult the person may become to live with. They are entering a reality that is much different from your own, beginning to see things much differently than you do.

They may become suspicious and believe that the items that keep going missing are being hidden or taken by others. There is little to be gained by trying to convince them otherwise. It may prove easier to simply agree with them and move along. You need to try and remember they are living in a different world than you are. This may take all the patience you can muster. Arguing rarely makes the situation better and may well make it worse.

My son bought me an electronic gadget to help me find things. The idea was to attach a little circular object to my keys, so when I couldn't find them, I could press a button on a device that would make the attachment buzz. Problem was, I kept losing the device.

My wife has said I used to assume that she knew what I was thinking about and that I started conversations totally out of context, expecting her to know what I was talking about when, in fact, I had given her no clue. When that happened, I, in turn, would get frustrated with what I perceived to be her lack of attention. The more you can honestly and clearly communicate with one another, the more you can enjoy each other's company. Unfortunately, clarity is at the top of the list of skills that diminish as dementia progresses.

Dr. Peter Rabins, at the John Hopkins Hospital in Baltimore, Maryland, has devoted much of his life to the study and treatment of Alzheimer's. With funding from the Jane Shapiro Family Education Program, the hospital has created a support center for family members that is named for and directed by Dr. Rabins. The following website will educate you about the disease and how to live with it. You will also find resources to make caregiving easier. www.hopkinsmedicine.org/psychiatry/specialty_areas/memory_center/rabinsalzheimers.

There is a video created by Dr. Rabins, which addresses many of the concerns I have been discussing. Much of what I learned about caregiving that I did not learn from my and my wife's experience or the partners and spouses of other cognitively impaired people, I learned from this website and others like it.

A web search will reveal a multitude of other sites that will provide a wide range of useful information and resources about dementia and caregiving. One of these is provided by AARP, the American Association of Retired Persons They have an online support center. If you visit www.arp.org/caregiving you will also find links to many topics of interest. Other websites I recommend you visit are www.alzheimers.acl.gov and www.eldercare.org, which will connect you with local organizations and services, and www.archrespite.org where you will learn about respite care, allowing you to have the occasional break from your caregiving responsibilities.

Taking Care of Yourself

Have you ever been on a plane? Always, before taking off, there is a safety briefing and you are told that, if and when the oxygen masks become necessary, to put on your own first. The point is obvious: you need to take care of yourself in order to be of help to anyone else.

There are some studies that have shown a direct relationship between caregiving and both emotional and physical health. The Spousal Caregivers of Dementia Victims: Longitudinal Changes in Immunity and Health Study was conducted at the Ohio State University College of Medicine in 1991. The authors tracked 69 spousal caregivers who, on average, had been caregiving for five years, and 69 socio-demographically matched control subjects for a period of thirteen months. They assessed changes in depression, immune function, and health. Their findings were quite informative. They found that over time caregivers showed a reduction of three measures of cellular immunity relative to control subjects. They reported significantly more days of infectious diseases, primarily upper respiratory infections, as well as a much greater incidence of depressive disorders. Interestingly enough, they also found that "caregivers who reported lower levels of social support at intake and who were distressed by dementia-related behaviors" showed the greatest and most uniformly negative changes in immune function at follow-up. Stress has been observed to be a risk factor in many diseases, including dementia. This study made it clear that the burden of caring for dementia patients can lead to emotional and physical illness.

Many books and articles have been written concerning the relationship between stress and deadly disease. Your own well-being, as well as the welfare of your loved one, depends on your staying both physically and mentally healthy. Very few things are as taxing as caring for someone with dementia. There are, however, strategies to deal with stress and it is very important you find some that work for you.

Recruiting a Team

There are so many tasks involved in caring for someone with dementia that no one person could possibly do it by themselves. Unfortunately, this sometimes happens at great cost to the well-being of the caregiver. Creating a team is essential for the primary caregiver and the patient. In addition to a number of healthcare professionals, this group will naturally include as many family members you can recruit, as well as friends. A family meeting should be called as soon as there is a diagnosis. If no diagnosis has been made, arrange a get together as soon as you realize there is a problem. If possible, the meeting should be held face-to-face. This will be an opportunity for everyone to become up-to-date on what is happening and what is likely to happen in the future. It will be a time to review the financial situation of the loved one as well as what expenses are likely to occur. You will have to decide who will assume responsibility for the hands-on care and who will be in charge of the finances. You may decide that multiple people will be filling some of these roles.

It needs to be agreed whose name will appear on bank accounts and who will be responsible for the timely payment of bills, and who will be entrusted with signing legal documents. It also needs to be determined what financial resources are available and to what extent people may wish to contribute to the costs of care. It may be wise to have double signatures required on some accounts to avoid disputes at a later date.

While it is a very good idea to hold the first meeting, and possibly the first several meetings, without the sick person present, once a basic plan has been formulated you will want your loved one to participate in a discussion of the strategy where their input can be sought.

The initial meetings will be the time to review what, if any, insurance policies are in place and is there a provision anywhere for long term care? The patient may be eligible for Social Security or retirement benefits. Recent legislation has made it possible for people with dementia in the U.S.A. to fast-track Social Security disability claims. Although I withdrew my first claim when I thought the problem had gone away, when I reopened it some months later, it was approved in less than six months.

A family meeting can also provide an opportunity for everyone involved to share his or her feelings and concerns. Sibling rivalries are often heightened at this critical time, and ex-partners and stepchildren can complicate the situation. It is essential to put aside any relationship conflicts to ensure that the best possible care is provided for your loved one. If this is proving difficult, there are therapists and mediators who are skilled in working with families of persons with dementia who find themselves in crisis and in need of guidance.

Hopefully, as the situation progresses, friends will come forward with offers of assistance, but you may need to ask. Be prepared to avail yourself of their support. Create a list of all the tasks that are involved in the day-to-day care of your loved one. This should include the myriad chores that are involved in managing a household. When someone asks if there is some way in which they can help, show them the list. It can include spending time with the person who is not well. Socializing is one of the things that can bring both meaning and joy into all our lives.

Do not be surprised if your friends are unable to see the extent of the problem. People with dementia have an amazing ability to appear perfectly normal for short periods of time. Add this to the fact that your friends are naturally going to want to think that their friend is fine and so there will be a lot of denial of the reality. Eventually, as the disease progresses, it will become increasingly obvious to them that your loved one is not well and that you are dealing with a difficult situation. It is most likely that your good friends will be more than willing to help.

Visits will be appreciated by the person who has dementia and, if the visitor agrees, can also create an opportunity for you to take a well-deserved break. As symptoms of dementia become more pronounced, friends may become reluctant to visit, afraid not only of the emotional pain of seeing someone they love suffering, but also questioning their own ability to help. Encourage them to keep visiting. It will be to everyone's advantage.

Speaking of breaks, it would be wise to investigate all possible means of taking them, as frequently as you can. If you belong to an organized religious group or fellowship, you may well find potential team members here. Many churches and synagogues have organized outreach programs for members who are ill. Even if you are not a member, there is no harm in inquiring. There may be adult day centers in your area, designed to provide a supervised setting for persons with cognitive impairment to spend the day. Such centers are usually open at least five days a week and may provide you with time for you to take care of yourself. In the United States, you should be able to find this information on www.archrespite.org and Alzheimer’s Associations everywhere will connect you with options for relief. Perhaps a family member could take over for a weekend while you take a mini-vacation. You deserve to have the best life possible during your time as a caregiver. Most of us have difficulty asking for help, but your well-being depends on having assistance, so be sure to ask family and friends to give you as much time as they can. It is a fact that caregivers who fail to or are unable to develop a support network are prone to more problems than those who do.

Support Groups

Probably one of the best strategies for dealing with the stress of caretaking is to join a support group. Participating in a group specifically for people who are providing care for, or care about, a person with dementia should be a part of any strategy for self-care whenever possible. Not only will you find emotional support, but hopefully you will also be exposed to a wealth of information about both the disease itself and the many resources available to you.

The value of connecting with others who understand exactly what you are going through cannot be overemphasized. You will receive encouragement and reassurance, and you will also be educated in every aspect of caring for your loved one. There are different types of groups, but they all have a common goal. That goal is to make your life as a caregiver more manageable.

It should not be too difficult to find one near you. If you visit the site www.alz.org, you will find information on those in your area. In addition to providing information about Alzheimer's, they also offer a 24/7 online message board where you will find additional support.

If you can't get out at all, or only occasionally, there are also online forums where you have the opportunity to ask questions, share information, and interact with other caregivers. Two are www.agingcare.com/caregiver and www.dementiaforum.org

Different groups follow different formats. Some have

professionals in the field of dementia who give talks. Others focus more on the sharing of experiences, and the emotions attached to them, while many offer a combination of the two. They will also provide you with fellowship, encouragement, and hope. Try to find the one that is right for you.

When looking for a support group, it is important to know the qualifications of the person or persons leading it. Ideally, they will be a professional who is trained in facilitating such groups. Experienced caregivers, however, also lead groups and can be of great help. Sharing your experiences, your frustrations and your fears with others that are going through the same thing somehow makes them feel less overwhelming as others identify with your challenges and struggles.

You will likely see people nodding their heads as if to say, "Me too." Not only will the feeling of being alone begin to dissipate, but you will also see that what you are feeling is normal. It is often very difficult for anyone who is not a caregiver to fully understand what you are going through. Here you will find empathetic ears. Listening to others share their experiences as caregivers is equally helpful. You may hear different approaches and strategies being shared that can be helpful to not only yourself but your loved one as well.

When you are new at caregiving, you will probably be unaware of the many opportunities to experience happiness, love, and joy that will present themselves during this time in your life. Listening to others share some of those experiences is sure to bring you hope.

Joining a support group is an easy way to add members to your team of people willing and able to help. While other members will surely be carrying their own heavy loads, it is very likely you will meet people willing to go for an occasional cup of coffee or chat on the phone.

It will be reassuring to know you are not alone, that all the feelings you are having are a normal part of the caregiving experience. You will also be given opportunities to ask questions, and the answers you receive will usually be given by people who have already done, or are doing, what you are trying to do.

Most groups meet at scheduled times and usually, but not always, they are held at times that don't conflict with work schedules. Some meet as often as twice a week, others biweekly and still others once a month. Once again, try to find a group that is right for you. You very well may make life-long friends in the process.

Sharing

One of the ways I try to avoid letting stress build up is to talk about things that are weighing heavily on my mind. In this process, several things happen. One is that my worries do not fester and overwhelm me. Another is that in the course of discussing situations with a trusted friend I may receive helpful feedback that opens up a new way of seeing things and may even lead to a solution or two. It seems that sometimes, left to my own devices I have difficulty in moving from the problem to a solution. If you do not have a friend in whom you can confide, you might consider a professional counselor. You may also find an empathetic ear at one of the agencies that offer care to caregivers.

I have also noticed that the more time I spend around other people, the less time I spend stressing out over my own problems. At the time when my symptoms were at their very worst, I had a friend who had much more advanced dementia than my own. His wife was not particularly adept at caretaking. Balls were being dropped, particularly in regard to doctors and medications. The more I was involved in helping him with his problems, his depression, and his fear, the less I thought about my own.

At one point, I arranged for him to visit the doctor I was seeing for my own problems. This doctor lived on a different island, and the trip took most of the day. I wrote down everything the doctor said because I knew my friend would not remember and I related the notes and instructions, including a new prescription, to his wife when we got home. I felt like I had made a difference. I could see him experiencing some hope for the first time in a while. The whole experience also made me feel better.

There is another benefit in trying to help someone else with their problem; it keeps my potential worst enemy, self-pity, at bay. There is no situation so dismal that self-pity cannot make it worse.

The awareness that the act of helping others could lift

my own spirits was the motivating factor for me to write this book. I am hoping that my experience of living with and recovering from dementia will be of value to others in a similar situation. The more I am concentrating on others, the less time I have to think about myself.

A guy named Bill Wilson and a doctor by the name of Bob Smith figured this same thing out over 80 years ago. That discovery became one of the cornerstones of recovery in what is now known as Alcoholics Anonymous. In fact, the last of the 12 steps, steps that have been adopted by millions as a way to find peace and serenity in the midst of despair, suggests that one help others overcome their problems. This program has been applied to dozens and dozens of illnesses other than alcoholism, and there is no reason why this concept shouldn't work for you.

Asking the person who has a full-time job caring for someone else to help others may at first seem counterintuitive and almost absurd. However, the more you involve yourself in the lives of others, the more you will find that everyone has their cross to bear, that we are all in this life together, and that together we can make it through anything. You are never alone.

Diet

A healthy diet, eaten at regular times, is also believed to reduce stress. And although having a cocktail or glass of wine will almost always take the edge off things that are bothering you, do not let your situation convince you that overindulgence is a good idea. It is not, and in fact, can often make tough times even worse.

The importance of a nutritious diet is stressed over and over in the ReCODE Protocol. As you have read in the chapter *How I am Recovering from Alzheimer's* proper nutrition is absolutely essential for a healthy mind. The protocol spells out quite clearly things to include and things to avoid to achieve a healthy metabolism. Although the suggestions regarding diet in the Protocol are directed at people with dementia, anyone can benefit from following them.

Being a caregiver can require physical and mental strength, both of which are supported by a healthy diet. Thankfully, eating well and eating simply go hand-in-hand. No complicated recipes are necessary. Fresh fruits and vegetables, lean meats and fish, lentils and beans and a minimum of processed foods are foundational to healthy nutrition. When preparing food, limit the amount of butter and fats and try to use olive oil. Check with your doctor about salt use, but generally less is best. Raw vegetables are a good choice, but if you want to cook them, then steaming is the way to go as more nutrients are retained.

If finding time to shop is a challenge, look for grocery stores in your community that will put together your order and deliver it to your home. When preparing meals, consider cooking double portions and freezing the extra to reheat on a day when you're too busy or don't have the energy to spend time in the kitchen.

Exercise

Another proven stress buster is exercise. Studies continue to confirm a definite correlation between exercise and not only mood but the level of cognitive functioning as well. Exercise can include running, working out at the gym, jogging or playing a team sport. It can also take the form of long walks and dancing. It's important to get your body moving and allow yourself to feel better physically and emotionally.

If at all possible, spend time outdoors. There is now a body of evidence indicating that exercising outdoors is even more effective and that spending time in nature will improve your well-being.

Work

If you are still working and the work is adding more stress to an already difficult situation, you might consider asking your boss or supervisor to rearrange some of your workload. Should you happen to be the boss, this could be the time to hone your delegation skills. If at all possible, you might consider promoting someone or increasing their compensation in exchange for easing some of your responsibilities. This is a time in your life when the idea of doing everything yourself has to be smashed. If it is impossible to rearrange your workload, and if you are not in a position to delegate some responsibilities, you might be well advised to consider finding a different job.

Sleep

Getting enough sleep is absolutely essential. Lack of

sufficient sleep has been associated with many health problems, including cognition. Research has shown that certain restorative processes in the brain happen only during deep sleep. The ReCODE Protocol addresses this subject, recommending a minimum of 8 hours sleep nightly. Stress makes getting sleep more difficult. So, does caring for someone whose internal clock has been upset, and is up throughout the night, but there are some solutions. If you are not getting enough sleep during the night, taking naps in the daytime can help ensure that your brain is getting enough downtime. Too many naps may exacerbate problems sleeping at night and should be kept to a healthy minimum.

Prescription medications can help provide short-term help with sleep, but their use must be closely monitored by your doctor as many of these lead to dependence and their own set of problems.

It has recently been discovered that spending time on computers or watching TV in the last hour before bed can have detrimental effects on sleep. It is also believed that setting consistent times for going to bed and awakening can help in the quest for healthier sleep patterns.

There are over-the-counter products available that can help. Melatonin has proven to be an effective non-pharmaceutical option for dealing with sleep deprivation and is available at almost any store that sells nutritional supplements. I have been using Melatonin for several years without any adverse effects, but side effects have been reported with its use, and it is best to talk to your doctor if you are considering taking it.

Meditation

Millions of people practice meditation on a daily basis, and its value in keeping stress levels low has been known for centuries. You don't need a guru, you don't need incense, and you don’t have to move to an ashram. Meditation can be practiced anywhere, although some people prefer to devote a space in their home for this to give themselves a retreat. A spare bedroom or den could work for this. There are many approaches to meditation, and one is not necessarily better than another. You need to find which way is best for you. Some people find sitting alone, with quiet, soothing music to be meditative. Others like to follow a guided meditation. These are available on CD, in music apps, as well as on YouTube. A web search of this topic will lead you to many websites.

Moving, or walking, meditation can include giving your full attention to the placement of your feet on the ground or to the mechanics of walking a dog. As the Buddhist monk, Thich Nhat Han, advises, when washing the dishes, wash the dishes. In other words, it is good to keep our attention on the task at hand and thereby calm the mind.

What seems to work for me is to simply sit quietly and try to calm the noise in my head. I have been practicing meditation for many years, and I cannot always achieve this stillness. There are, however, things I can do to help. One of these is to keep focusing on my breathing.

Whenever I find myself drifting back to busy or worry mode, I go back to concentrating on my breath. Sometimes, I imagine myself breathing out fear on my exhale and taking in positive virtues like love and faith on the inhaling breath. As I breathe in, I say, "love" and as I exhale "fear." Find for yourself the things you want more or less of. I do not always use fear and love, sometimes I use anger and acceptance.

I encourage you to give it a try and keep it simple. You can start with five minutes and build your meditation time slowly. However, it has been shown that a minimum of 20 minutes is most beneficial. Whatever amount of time you choose, if you achieve five or ten minutes of real inner calm, you have succeeded. And if on occasion this doesn't happen, remember there is no failure in meditation, there is only practice. And, for however long you sat, for just that much time was your body at rest, which is restorative in itself. I have found that the more I practice, the more I am able to give my mind a rest from its incessant chatter. There are hundreds of books, videos and instruction manuals to help you get started.

Mindfulness-Based Stress Reduction (MBSR) is an eight-week course offered in almost every major city in North America and has brought a new sense of peace and a new way of coping into the lives of countless people. Developed by Jon Kabat-Zin, the author of a very helpful book, Full Catastrophe Living, the program, taught by trained leaders, has been the subject of numerous studies, which have shown it to be effective in reducing stress, enhancing relaxation and improving quality of life. To find an MBSR program near you, go to the website www.umasmed.edu/cfm/mindfulness-based-programs/mbsr-courses/find-an-mbsr-program or search MBSR and your city name online.

The Alzheimer Research and Prevention Foundation has endorsed another form of meditation, which enhances, among other things, brain fitness and memory, and reduces stress. Kirtan Kriya can be best described as a singing meditation. You don't need to have a singing voice though, as the tune is simple and there are only four words to remember: Saa taa naa maa. With the palm extended, the thumb and three fingers, starting with the index, are touched to the pointer finger one at a time while saying one of the words. Attention is focused on the L formed when the fingers meet and on the pressure at the fingertips. For two minutes you sing in a normal voice, then sing in a hushed voice for the next four minutes and finally say the words to yourself. If you'd like to learn more about Kirtan Kriya, you can visit www.alzheimersprevention.org and choose "yoga".

Just remember, the purpose of meditation is to relax and free your mind from the flotsam and jetsam that clutters the space between our ears.

Yoga

People all over the world practice yoga on a daily basis, in its many forms. Some yoga practices are quite physically demanding, and some are quite gentle.

Whatever type of yoga you practice, it will reduce your stress, help you feel more relaxed and improve your physical well-being. As with meditation, you do not need a guru, incense or an ashram. Although many people prefer to do yoga in a group setting, with a teacher guiding the movements, it is not essential. In fact, you do not even have to take a class if time or money do not permit. There are dozens, if not hundreds, of DVD's that can teach you what you need to get started.

My wife did yoga at home in front of a tape playing on the TV for years. She now practices without a tape as she has learned all of the poses she needs to know. Although certain situations, like moving back and forth from the Caribbean, will stress her out, for the most part, she is one of the most relaxed people that I know. You can also find many instructional yoga videos online. Just type in “yoga” on Google or any other search engine, and you are sure to find one. When I was running a large business, I used to start every workday with a yoga posture known as the Sun Salutation. It took less than a minute of my time, but it helped me start the day with a positive attitude. Many physicians believe that stress is at the root of a significant percentage of backaches and the physical strain of providing care can also result in backache. There are numerous yoga poses that could alleviate your pain.

If you believe that yoga is too difficult or too time-consuming, this would be the right time to try to have an open mind and remind yourself of the potential benefits.

Caregivers need all the help they can get.

The Emotional Freedom Technique

The Emotional Freedom Technique (EFT), developed in the 1990s by Gary Craig has demonstrated success in reducing both stress and depression. Proponents of this technique believe that tapping your fingers on certain places on your body known as meridian points, while simultaneously verbalizing custom-made affirmations, can reprogram the way your body responds to stressors. This technique can be facilitated by a trained therapist or can also be done on your own. A web search will give you lots of information and, if you decide to practice EFT without a therapist, you can find several videos demonstrating how to perform this technique. It is, however, highly recommended that for optimum results you work with a therapist, especially in the beginning

Guilt, Self-Pity and the Antidote

An emotion that often adds to higher stress levels is feelings of guilt. At all times you must remember that you are performing a herculean task and that you are doing the best you can in a very trying situation. Try to remember to acknowledge that to yourself frequently. You are a hero.

Well-meaning friends will probably be offering suggestions from time to time on how to care for your loved one. Occasionally, these comments may seem to be critical of the way you are doing things. Try to remember that they are trying to be helpful and that their suggestions are more than likely to be coming from a place of very little knowledge or experience. And once again, try to remain open-minded, as some of these suggestions may prove quite helpful.

Equally as dangerous as stress can be the feeling of self-pity. Taking care of a sick person full-time changes everything. If you are the primary caregiver, it will require an enormous amount of your time. Your social life will change as your schedule becomes more and more dedicated to the patient. It will become increasingly difficult to leave your loved one alone. There may seem to be precious little time for yourself, let alone socializing.

That feeling of "Why me?" or worse, "Poor me" is bound at some point to appear. Those types of feelings, if allowed to fester, can lead straight to depression, a disease in its own right. Should that happen, and it often does, remember that serious, clinical depression many times does not go away of its own accord. You would be well advised to seek the help of a physician if you find yourself in that situation.

When my dementia was at its worst, I believed my condition was fatal. I knew myself well enough to know that if I allowed myself to start feeling sorry for myself, my remaining years would be miserable.

I avoided self-pity like the plague. One way I did this was by trying to maintain an attitude of gratitude at all times and it is the best antidote for self-pity. So, how do you remain grateful in the midst of serious difficulty? I can tell you how I did. It was a combination of many things in no particular order of importance. Even though I was certain at the time that I would be dead in a few years, I felt like at least I had time to get my affairs in order, as best I could. I reminded myself regularly that the world was full of people who had much, much worse problems than I did. I was living in one of the most prosperous countries on earth, and I had all the creature comforts that go with that. I knew that I was living in a country where it was very easy to keep up with any breakthroughs in the treatment of dementia. Interestingly enough, I did not learn of Dr. Bredesen's work with his protocol while living in a U.S. Territory, but I was very fortunate to learn of the protocol while living in Mexico, by way of some American friends.

I also was very much aware of the fact that I had a wife who would stick by my side no matter what and would never let harm come to me. Also, I have been blessed with many friends. I was able to talk about my situation in depth with a select few of them. In times of crisis, it is easy to see who your real friends are, and I am grateful for every one of them that I have.

As I mentioned earlier, I had a close friend who was much sicker than me and was not getting the kind of support that I was. Seeing his situation made me very grateful for the support that I was receiving. It also reaffirmed the fact that many others were in worse circumstances than me. How could I feel sorry for myself when my friend was in a much worse situation than me?

Try and imagine how fortunate your loved one is to

have a person like you at her side, and what an awesome thing it is that she has entrusted you with keeping her safe and attended to. Can you be grateful that you have the love, courage, patience, and fortitude to accomplish that task? Feel free to give yourself lots of pats on the back. You deserve them!

There are many wonderful things in all of our lives that we tend to take for granted. Take the time to consider these things, and you will see that despite the trying circumstances you are in, you are a very fortunate person.

My friend and editor, India Taylor, worked for many years in the field of elder care and has taught classes on nurturing an attitude of gratitude. She has agreed to contribute some of her thoughts on the subject:

"Gratitude can be both an easy and challenging practice. Often you may feel as though there is nothing to be thankful for. When your partner or friend is diagnosed with dementia, when you have sleepless nights followed by days of multiple medical appointments, when you are exhausted and angry it may seem impossible to find one thing for which you can be grateful. I know, I've been there. But if you allow yourself a few moments of reflection, you may be surprised at what you can think of. It's not necessary to have "big" items on your gratitude list. A roof over your head, food in the fridge, caring doctors and taps that don't leak are all excellent reasons to give thanks. Research shows that practicing gratitude can improve your physical and mental health, build

strong relationships and even help you sleep better. It's called a gratitude practice because its best for us to make it a regular part of our day - a regular practice, like brushing your teeth. It's recommended that you journal the things you are thankful for; pick three to five things. Reviewing these when you are having a hard day may prove to be helpful. It can focus you on the positives in your life. It's also good to express gratitude to the people in your life. You could write a thank you note, phone someone to express your appreciation or share a hug. Cultivating gratitude takes little time but can yield large results."

There is one more thing that should help you to remain upbeat. You are reading this book. In it, you will learn of many patients that have managed to recover from dementia. If your loved one has not advanced so far in the disease that recovery is no longer possible, you will find everything you need to know to begin the recovery process.

Wisdom from my Wife

My wife, Patricia, has reminded me of a few of her favorite stress-busting techniques. She loves to read, and we all know an interesting book can take us to places far removed from our trouble and turmoil. Becoming absorbed in a really good plot, regardless of what it is, is sure to take you away from the worries you have at home. If you have gotten out of the habit of reading, now is a good time to return to it. If you have never developed the habit of reading for pleasure, give it a try. Ask some friends for their recommendations until you hear of a novel, collection of short stories or biography that appeals to you and, if they have a copy, ask if you can borrow it. A web search might also steer you to some entertaining comics. This genre has come a long way in recent years, and some levity may be just what the doctor ordered.

In the public library, you will find not only great books but also a haven of peace and quiet. It may have book groups, and there may also be some in your community that are organized by friends or organizations. Many towns and all cities have groups that meet regularly to discuss the books they are reading. Ask around, and you will probably be able to find one. They are free, and they will provide you with an opportunity to socialize and take your mind off of other worries.

Another thing my wife believes is very helpful in the war against stress is therapeutic massage. We live in Mexico, and we are very fortunate. A fully trained massage therapist will bring her table to our house and do a complete 75-minute massage for around 35 dollars. She will usually bring a tape player with very relaxing music and for the time she is there my wife will be in a different world.

The first time I was leaving a massage appointment, it took me several minutes to figure out why I felt so different. I was simply not accustomed to not having 50 pounds of stress sitting on my shoulders. While a professional massage may well cost more where you are, there are many massage therapists that have a sliding scale fee structure. Call several if you have to until you find one that fits your budget. I think you will be glad that you did! There may be a school of massage in your town and, if so, give them a call as they usually offer massages with students at great rates.

My wife is also very fond of Tai Chi. Like yoga, Tai Chi can be practiced at home alone and requires no special equipment. Passed down from ancient Chinese traditions, some people like to call it meditation in motion. Through a series of exercises and stretches that flow one into another, your body is kept in slow and gentle motion. It is a graceful form of exercise that has been providing health benefits to millions of people all over the world for centuries. Three benefits are increased energy and strength, improvement in the symptoms of depression, and the reduction of stress. Sounds like just what the doctor ordered, doesn't it?

If you are interested in exploring Tai Chi, it would be best to begin by taking a class with a qualified instructor. By doing so you will not only learn the proper technique, but you will also be advised which moves to avoid that might aggravate any existing physical conditions you may have. You can find a class by inquiring at gyms and health clubs or by contacting a senior’s center near you. And, like almost always, a web search can assist you in finding a class nearby. If a classroom introduction is not feasible, there are numerous sites online that can direct you towards books,

DVDs and other sources of information on Tai Chi.

There is a helpful DVD, published in November 2014, entitled Top 10 Tai Chi Moves for Beginners, which is available on YouTube, courtesy of The Kung Fu and Tai Chi Center with Jake Mace. As promised, the video offers a demonstration of ten of the best movements for a beginner at Tai Chi. The video is slow paced and repetitive and easy to follow. You just might find this practice becoming a part of your stress buster tool kit.

Move a Muscle, Change a Thought

One last suggestion can be summarized in six simple words: “move a muscle, change a thought”. I first heard this expression many years ago, and I have been employing it ever since.

I used to have a chair I called my “thinking chair.” It was very comfortable. It became my favorite place to sit and ponder the state of the world. Unfortunately, as often as not, during the time when I was suffering from dementia, my thinking would become centered on myself and, in truth, it became my “worrying chair”. After hearing that six-word expression, I began to notice that if I got tired of worrying, or if I couldn’t stop myself from negative thinking, the simple act of getting out of the chair and moving into the next room almost always got my mind on a different subject, usually a benign one. Sometimes just getting up and washing my hands achieved the same result.

As I hope you can see, there are many ways to deal with the stress of caring for a loved one that is seriously ill, and I am certain I have not mentioned all of them. My wife has told me over and over, that I need to mention that taking a bath can do wonders. So, I am mentioning it now.

Whichever way you find to deal with stress, it is extremely important that you do so, as stress-related behavior and illness can be quite damaging to both yourself and your loved one.

IT'S NOT ALWAYS ALZHEIMER'S

When I first started having more serious problems with memory, the kind that started to scare me, my mind went immediately to the Big A. I knew nothing about it, could not even spell it, but I was totally convinced I had it.

I don't remember exactly when I decided to get medical help and go to a doctor. All I know for sure is that I waited too long. But I finally went, and when I kept insisting I had Alzheimer's, I must have driven the guy crazy. It took many visits with him before I finally understood that a person could have Mild Cognitive Impairment (MCI), or even actual dementia, and not have the disease I was so certain I had. I am sure when I first started seeing the doctor, he was right, I had MCI.

I had a hard time accepting the diagnosis of Mild Cognitive Impairment. I did not know it was a condition that may or may not eventually lead to full-blown Alzheimer's. There was nothing about my situation that felt mild to me. Had I been capable of adequately describing the things that were happening to me, the doctor's job would probably have been much easier. It is a very good idea to have a spouse or a close friend accompany you on visits to the doctor. If not, there is a good chance you will not be giving a full report on your condition, and you are very likely to forget at least some of the things you are being told as well as things you want to say. If you are given a diagnosis of MCI or actual dementia ... DO NOT PANIC.

Dementia is not a specific disease. It is an umbrella term that covers many sub-types, all of which affect mental ability to the degree that it impacts on daily life, affecting memory, thinking, and social abilities. According to the Mayo Clinic, in order to make a diagnosis of dementia, there must be problems with at least two separate brain functions, such as:

- Memory loss greater than that of normal aging
- Impaired judgment and language problems
- Inability to perform daily activities, like paying bills or driving without getting lost.

Dementia has many symptoms, not all of which may manifest. Common symptoms include problems with memory, changes in personality, inability to recall common words, agitation, strange behaviors, difficulty reasoning, and even hallucinations.

The biggest problem for me was my inability to remember not only events that were happening but also things I was supposed to be doing. Trying to get ready to leave the house became a major process, and often I would not remember to buckle my pants and zip up my fly before going out the door. I would get extremely agitated when I could not find things, which was constantly, and I would pay for things in stores and then walk out, leaving them behind. There were many other things happening all day long that were making my life difficult, but I think you have the idea.

Mild Cognitive Impairment is often the first stage of dementia. Most, but not all, persons with MCI progress to dementia at some point, and 70 percent of them will eventually develop Alzheimer's. If you have already been diagnosed with MCI, DO NOT ASSUME THE WORST. I eventually learned there were many different types of cognitive impairment. I would have been aware of that sooner if I had not spent so much time arguing with my doctor.

I also discovered that some forms of cognitive decline are REVERSIBLE, that it is not always a one- way street to institutionalization. In fact, recent studies are offering convincing evidence that almost all types of dementia are reversible to some extent.

One thing I gleaned from my experience is that people with cognitive impairment are reluctant to study things that are new or complicated. The brain does not like to be confronted with its inadequacies. It is too painful. For that reason, while most of the information available on dementia is highly scientific in nature, my intention is to share what I have learned without going too much into the science of it.

Much of what I have learned is available on the internet, but when I was at the low point of my cognitive abilities, even doing a simple web search was too much for me. Sometimes, turning on the computer seemed too much.

I hope the information I am providing, while no way 100 percent complete, will give the reader a basic understanding of what may be going on with people experiencing memory difficulties and what can be done about it.

Reversible Cognitive Impairment

Please bear in mind that the information presented here about reversible forms of dementia is based on science that predates Dr. Bredesen's on reversing Alzheimer's itself.

If I had known there were several types of cognitive impairment that were reversible, I am certain I would have investigated them at the first signs of trouble. But once again, I knew nothing and thought I knew everything, so I did not. Perhaps this unwillingness to be open to new information was itself a part of the impairment. As I think about it, it must have been. All my life I had been inquisitive by nature, excited about learning new things. Until then.

The most frequent potentially reversible causes of cognitive impairment are:

•Drugs (can be any drug with anticholinergic activity)

- Alcohol abuse
- Depression
- Nutritional conditions (vitamin deficiency)
- Stress
- Hyperthyroidism
- Normal pressure hydrocephalus

Anticholinergic Drugs

"Anticholinergic" refers to a class of drugs that affect the smooth muscles of the body and are used to treat sleep disorders, depression, and incontinence among other things. With the exception of Nyquil, they can be found in almost all of the night-time over-the-counter medications. Unfortunately, their use can result in dementia-like symptoms.

While the link between these anticholinergics and cognitive decline has been known for years, the cognitive decline associated with these drugs has until recently thought to be reversible upon discontinuation of their use. Current studies have now discovered convincing evidence of a link between anticholinergic drugs and what has until lately been considered irreversible dementia. In a study published in JAMA Internal Medicine (formerly Archives of Internal Medicine), titled "Cumulative Use of Strong Anticholinergics and Incident Dementia" (Eric Lawson, Shelly L. Gray et. al, University of Washington, 2015), a definite correlation between use of these drugs and a later incidence of dementia was found.

The study included 3,434 participants, none of who

displayed any symptoms of dementia at the study's start. They found that the most common anticholinergic classes used were tricyclic antidepressants and first-generation, older, antihistamines. The researchers found that after follow-ups averaging 7.3 years, 23.2 percent of the participants had developed dementia. Of these, 79.9 percent had gone on to develop Alzheimer's. They concluded that the higher the cumulative use of these drugs, the greater the risk of developing dementia and or Alzheimer's.

Obviously, there is a need for physicians to be looking for substitutes for these medications wherever possible. If you are taking any of these drugs, the sooner you can find an alternative the better.

If you are not sure that you are taking these meds, the online site www.agingbrain.org has a chart that will give you the common names of all of them. If you are taking any of these drugs it is absolutely IMPERATIVE that you INFORM YOUR DOCTOR.

Depression

It's important to remember that cognitive impairment is not the same thing as dementia. It can be a precursor to dementia, but not always.

A 1990 article in the Indian Journal of Psychiatry reported a study that found 18 percent of all dementia stemmed from potentially reversible conditions. For this reason, it is CRITICAL that tests be done early and thoroughly.

In May of 2013, the New York Times published an

article that had appeared in the British Journal of Psychiatry a few days earlier. The study was based on an analysis of over 50,000 adults that collectively had participated in a total of 23 separate studies on dementia.

They found that depressed older adults (defined as those over the age of fifty) were more than TWICE AS LIKELY to develop vascular dementia and 65 percent MORE LIKELY to develop Alzheimer's disease than similarly aged people who were not depressed.

It is not surprising that my doctor chose to pursue this line of investigation first. He told me that he strongly suspected that I was depressed the first time I was in his office.

We treated the depression with a combination of medication and talk therapy. After a few months, I was beginning to experience joy and happiness for the first time in years and the depression was lifting. Unfortunately, my cognitive decline continued to progress.

A study, published in 2000, in The Journal of the American Geriatrics, reported on following 111 subjects with cognitive impairment, but no neurological or somatic causes for that impairment, for five years. By the end of the follow-up, 25 of the subjects had preclinical dementia with Alzheimer's type dementia. Of these, 60 percent had reported being seriously depressed at the start of the study.

Although there is no definite proof that depression causes impairment, there is obviously a clear link between the two. Since depression can be treated with a number of different medicines, as well as talk therapy, seeking professional help will not only hopefully relieve you of the depression, it may improve your cognitive ability, while at the same time improve your chances of not developing dementia later.

Stress

It is no news to anyone that stress can have a negative influence on the body. It should come as no surprise that there is now a wealth of data linking stress with negative effects on the mind. There are hundreds of studies that connect stress to health issues. It reduces the immune function, it can lead to high blood pressure, and it can disrupt hormone balance. The lack of sleep that so often accompanies stress can lead to other complications. And cognitive function is one of them.

Recent research seems to suggest that stress is also related to the onset of Alzheimer's disease itself. Given the relative ineffectiveness of existing medication for dementia and the fact that as yet there is no "proven" cure for Alzheimer's, other than the ReCODE Protocol the need for preventive measures is of paramount importance for anyone beginning to show symptoms of cognitive decline. Stress reduction will not only lead to a more pleasant life; it may very well prolong it.

Dr. Edgardo Reich recently reported to the World Conference of Neurology his findings on the relationship between stress and the clinical onset of Alzheimer's disease. He said, "Stress, according to our findings, is probably a trigger for initial symptoms of dementia." He went on to say, "Though I rule out stress as mono-causal in dementia, research is solidifying the evidence that stress can trigger a degenerative process in the brain..."

Dr. Reich's study, conducted in Argentina, found that nearly three out of four (72 percent) Alzheimer's patients had experienced severe emotional stress during the two years preceding their diagnosis. In the control group, only one out of four had experienced major stress or grief during the same period. Once again, while no one is saying that stress will definitely cause dementia, there is a clear relationship between the two.

Much has been written about how to reduce the stress in your life. It is well known that a great deal of stress is work related and that there are many ways to reduce it. There are books on the subject in every bookstore. There is even a program that utilizes "energy psychology techniques." Developed by Gary Craig, the technique is known as EFT and involves tapping parts of the body in conjunction with verbal affirmations.

The techniques that work best for me are exercise, yoga, and meditation. When I was no longer able to successfully operate my business, I had no choice other than to retire. This by itself released a huge amount of stress, and my wife was commenting on improvements in my memory very shortly after we moved to Mexico. If you are suffering from stress, you owe it to yourself to seek out ways to reduce it and practice them.

If I had eliminated both stress and depression from my

life fifteen years ago, I honestly believe my life would be very different today.

Vitamin Deficiency

Vitamin deficiency is one of the more common causes of reversible cognitive impairment. It is also the easiest one to test for. A simple trip to the local blood lab can confirm or discount this possibility. If you live in the United States, you will, of course, need a physician to order the tests. In many countries, however, you can simply go to the lab and order it yourself.

However, by now you should have a working relationship with at least one doctor. If not, you are making a terrible mistake. Today one of the major components of the ReCODE Protocol is individualized testing for all aspects of nutrition. The nutritional supplements I take on a daily basis are for me one of the most critical components of rigorously practicing the Protocol.

I did have blood work done to see if I had any vitamin deficiencies. While there was evidence of minor anemia, there was nothing to suggest dementia. I should have also had tests done to determine if there was any blockage of blood flow to the brain, but, for financial reasons, I did not.

Eventually, I did have a CT scan performed, but again the test revealed nothing. Unfortunately, deeply entrenched thinking in the medical community upholds that other types of dementia are both untreatable and fatal. Hence there appears to be reluctance, once the potentially reversible dementias are ruled out, to not spend much time differentiating what type of illness might be causing the symptoms. At least that was my experience.

Interestingly enough, 45 percent of Alzheimer's patients and their caregivers report that they had never been given a formal diagnosis. This may be a result of hesitancy on the part of medical professionals to offer a diagnosis for a disease that is considered fatal, or it may be the result of the patient's failure to follow through with enough testing to give an accurate diagnosis. The more that scientists clarify the importance of treating the symptoms of Alzheimer's as early as possible, this will no doubt change. The sooner all these tests are performed, the better the chances for a positive outcome, so once again, DO NOT DELAY!

TYPICAL PROGRESSION OF DEMENTIA

Dementia is a broad category of brain diseases that cause long-term and often gradual decreases in the ability to think and remember such that a person's daily life is affected. In the fifth edition of the Diagnostic and Statistical Manual of Mental Disorders (DSM 5), dementia was reclassified as a neurocognitive disorder with varying degrees of severity.

It is believed that approximately 10 percent of the general population will develop the disease at some point in their lives. The likelihood of developing dementia grows as people age. Almost 80 percent of people in their 80s have the disease.

Early Stage

Although MCI (Mild Cognitive Impairment) isn’t considered full-blown dementia, often it is the first visible stage of dementia. As mentioned earlier, approximately 70 percent of the time MCI progresses to dementia, but not always.

Mild Cognitive Impairment can be described as an intermediary phase between normal cognitive decline associated with aging and the onset of dementia. In the early stages, changes are just beginning to become apparent. Signs of cognitive decline will begin to be noticeable to the people closest to the person as well as those he interacts with on a regular basis.

There will be observable changes in memory. Other symptoms may include an occasional inability to find the right word, difficulty finding things like keys and purses that have misplaced, and forgetting to take medications.

Although forgetful and somewhat disorganized, people in this stage are capable of taking care of themselves. They may repeat themselves or forget to take their medicine, but their lives are still manageable.

In this early stage, organizational skills are just beginning to show impairment. An inability to manage finances often manifests at the end of this stage and difficulties in the workplace become noticeable.

In my case, for a long time, no one was paying any attention to my finances but me. My wife had been experiencing her own cognitive difficulties for quite some time, and the area of finance was strictly my domain.

Here was an area where once again my ego prevented me from seeking help. Part of me was in denial about the state of my finances, always believing that they would soon be better. I had no desire for anyone to know that my business was losing money, including myself. So, I did not seek help, and the deterioration continued.

My wife suspected something was amiss before anyone else did, but she did not know what. She repeatedly told me I was making bad decisions, but I kept assuming she didn't understand the business model. She was definitely aware I was using our own money to make payroll on a regular basis and commented multiple times that something was wrong. In my mind, these were short-term loans, soon to be paid back. They never were.

Someone once told me that there are situations where "you can't save your ass and your face at the same time." This was one of those situations. I absolutely should have been listening to my wife, but my thinking was too impaired to see that. That is one of the problems with cognitive impairment and dementia in general. Your brain is not seeing what it is not seeing.

One thing I can tell you with certainty is that by the time MCI is firmly entrenched, there is nothing mild about it. It is true that many who suffer from MCI will not progress further, but most do.

Middle Stage

In the middle stage of dementia, symptoms worsen, and this phase can go on for many years. It becomes very difficult, and eventually impossible, for the memory to retain any new information. It is also becoming increasingly difficult to participate in many types of social interactions. Faces and names will not be remembered, and social settings will have become increasingly uncomfortable.

There will be an inability to manage most of one's affairs. Important decisions of any kind will need to be made by others. Eventually, assistance will be required for personal care and hygiene.

Easily agitated, people in this stage become increasingly burdensome on caregivers. The caregivers themselves will often start experiencing health problems of their own. This phase may go on for as long as six or seven years, though there are cases where the duration of middle stage dementia has gone on longer.

Late Stage

The final stage of dementia, also referred to as advanced or severe dementia, has always been thought to result in the need for 24-hour care. Often, those with late stage dementia do not want to get out of bed. Eventually, they become incapable of doing so, they become incontinent, and they lose the capacity for speech.

At this point, patients withdraw from all the things that make life worth living. They no longer recognize most of the people who are closest to them and the will to live, to participate in the ebb and flow of life, is gone, slowly evaporated. All appetite is lost, the organs shut down, and that is the end.

The race to find a cure for dementia is in full swing. There are research centers all over the world trying to find the answer or answers to this heartbreaking riddle. It is only in the last several years that any success in reversing or delaying the progression of dementia has been reported. Now, for the first time, THERE IS HOPE for people with the disease. I know this for a fact because the progression of my disease has been halted.

In the following chapters, I will provide an overview of the different kinds of dementia.

NON-ALZHEIMER'S DEMENTIAS

Vascular Dementia

Vascular Dementia, after Alzheimer's, is the leading cause of dementia, responsible for 20 percent of all cases. It is caused by disease or injury to the blood vessels and impairs blood flow to the brain. The brain needs the vitamins and minerals found in the blood to function properly. When the flow is impeded, damage occurs.

According to Carrie Hill, PhD., who has spent years studying and working hands-on with dementia patients, between one and four percent of people over the age of 65 have vascular dementia. The chances of developing it increase dramatically as one ages.

It was originally believed that this type of dementia was caused solely by either one major stroke or a series of smaller ones. It is now known that there is a whole host of medical conditions and diseases that are capable of inhibiting the flow of blood to the brain. Several factors have been identified as putting a person more at risk for vascular dementia.

The following conditions are often found in the histories of those with this disease:

- Heart Attack
- High Cholesterol
- High Blood Pressure
- Diabetes
- Stroke

Not every person that has a stroke will develop dementia, but approximately one-third of them will do so in less than a year after having had it. It does not take a major stroke for this to happen. A series of small strokes can have the same result, with the possibility of developing the disease closely correlated with the number of such events.

Symptoms

The presence of vascular dementia can manifest in a variety of ways. In addition to memory problems, there is likely to be problems with executive functioning. The ability for strategic thinking and planning, the ability to manage finances, and the ability to maintain social relationships may all be seriously impaired. Unfortunately, these symptoms also occur in other types of dementia.

Some symptoms, however, are specific to vascular dementia. One of these can be the presence of exaggerated reflexes. There will also be neurological problems, including weakness in the hands, limbs, and feet, difficulty maintaining one's balance, and abnormal gait. Delusions, depression, and agitation may also be found in this type of dementia. One thing that differentiates Vascular Dementia from Alzheimer's is a more rapid onset of symptoms. Another is the fact that some, but not necessarily all, cognitive functions will be impaired.

Unlike Alzheimer's, the first symptoms to appear will often be the neurological ones. Also, unlike Alzheimer's, the progression of the disease is not a consistent. downward trajectory. Rather, the patient will vacillate between periods of stability and periods of decline. The transition between times of stability and those of inability to function effectively can be sudden and dramatic.

As with all types of dementia, the presence of any or all of these symptoms should be IMMEDIATELY REPORTED to your doctor, who will do a complete diagnostic workup. This will usually include ordering procedures to detect the presence of narrowing or blockage of the arteries, as well as to look for evidence of strokes. These procedures will be accompanied by cognition tests, some of which can be performed right in the doctor's office, to evaluate the extent of cognitive decline.

The diagnosis of any type of dementia will include the ruling out of all other possible causes for the symptoms being presented.

Treatment

The FDA has to date approved no medications for the treatment of Vascular Dementia, but some of the medicines that have been approved for use in treating Alzheimer's can sometimes be effective in managing the symptoms of Vascular Dementia. Medications like Aricept and Exelon have proven beneficial for patients with vascular dementia.

In the presence of this type of dementia, it is very important to keep an eye on blood pressure, cholesterol, and blood sugar, as these are known to be directly related to the ability of blood to flow to the brain freely.

Recent studies are showing beyond a doubt that there is a direct correlation between lifestyle and brain health. Changes to diet and way of living can make dramatic differences.

Lewy Body Dementia

In 1912, while studying the brains of people with Parkinson's disease, Dr. Frederick Lewy, a German-born neurologist who moved to the U.S. during World War Two, discovered the presence of abnormal protein deposits in the mid-section of these brains. Then, in the 1960s, these deposits, now referred to as Lewy bodies, were found to exist not only in the mid-section but also in the cortex of the brains of some people with dementia. That category of patients has what is now called Lewy Body Dementia (LBD).

These Lewy bodies are only visible during an autopsy, and since the symptoms of this disease are so similar to Alzheimer's, it often goes undiagnosed or misdiagnosed. It is also possible for a person with LBD to suffer from other dementias, most commonly Alzheimer's.

Symptoms

Unlike the other types of dementia, symptoms in people with LBD can vary from person to person and from day to day. The symptoms seem to mimic both Alzheimer's and the motor problems typical of Parkinson's disease.

A definite diagnosis of LBD is, at present, impossible to make while the patient is still alive, although tests can be done post-mortem to do so. It is often difficult to distinguish this disease from Alzheimer's, however, there is one symptom that is more characteristic of LBD than any other type of dementia. This is the development of both cognitive decline and motor difficulties within a year of one another, with the motor difficulties usually manifesting first. Other symptoms include:

- Visual and Non-Visual hallucinations
- Loss of inhibition, socially or sexually inappropriate behavior
- Depression
- Delusions
- Fainting
- Frequent Falls

The severity and presence of symptoms can vary from day to day. The person may be functioning fine for a period of time, only to be followed by another decline.

A definitive diagnosis of LBD is still only possible at death; however, physicians can make a clinical diagnosis based on a medical history, test results and the symptoms you report. It is imperative to remember, once again, that you have to REPORT YOUR SYMPTOMS. THE SOONER THE BETTER.

Treatment

Although at present there is no recognized cure for LBD, the standard treatment is to try to alleviate the symptoms associated with it. The depression that often accompanies the disease is treatable with medication, and there are other drugs, such as Aricept, Razadyne, and Reminyl, that have been shown to help with not only cognitive decline but also with the hallucinations that often come with LBD. None of these treatments can delay the progression of the disease; they merely alleviate the symptoms.

People with LBD sometimes exhibit aggressive behavior. This behavior, especially when out of character, can be both challenging and upsetting to family, friends, and caregivers. The aggression may result from infections, untreated pain or other unmet needs. I believe this aggression may also stem from the fear and anxiety they experience as a result of not being able to control or share their reality, which often is very different from our own. Patients believe the hallucinations they are seeing are real, and when others try to tell them they are not, it arouses fear and anger. The best course of action is to not argue, and rather, focus on relieving their discomfort.

In the end stages of the disease, the treatment will be centered on managing the physical deterioration that will occur, including increasingly impaired motor skills that may result in broken bones, stiffness and rigidity that make movement very difficult, sleep difficulties, and ever-increasing hallucinations. The caregiver's job is becoming increasingly difficult.

Prognosis

Historically the prognosis has been as follows. LBD will progress slowly over time. Death usually occurs between five and seven years after the first arrival of symptoms. It is known to occur, however, as early as two years and as long as twenty years after that. Death usually results from either pneumonia or any one of a number of different infections. Other frequently observed causes of death are complications related to falling.

Frontotemporal Dementia

Frontotemporal Dementia (FTD) is the name of a group of disorders that are caused by the progressive deterioration of nerve cells in the brain's frontal lobes (the area behind the forehead), or it's temporal lobes (the region behind the ears). These are the areas of the brain that control emotions, the capacity for judgment and planning, speaking as well as comprehending speech, and certain types of motor skills.

Once considered to be a rare form of dementia, it is now, according to the American Alzheimer's Association website www.alz.org, believed to account for as many as 15 percent of dementia cases. Among persons under the age of 65 with dementia, FTD is thought to account for approximately 50 percent of them.

The ages at which people are affected by FTD tells us

that dementia is not always an “old person’s” disease. FTD often develops in the 50s and 60s, but it can happen as early as the 20s.

There are three main categories of disorders that comprise FTD. Please do not let the scientific nature of the words that follow discourage you. The disorders are easier to understand than they are to pronounce.

Behavior Variant FTD

Of the three disorders, Behavior Variant FTD (bvFTD) is the one that accounts for the most pronounced changes in personality and behavior. In the beginning stages of this type of FTD, the symptoms will mimic those of Alzheimer's. As the disease progresses, however, the patient will usually begin to exhibit an obvious lack of restraint in their personal relations and their social life will begin to be characterized by incidents of inappropriate actions.

There are many symptoms of bvFTD that are common to other types of dementia, such as apathy, changes in personal hygiene and problems with memory. It is the profound changes in personality and conduct that sets bvFTD apart.

Primary Progressive Aphasia

This category of FTD affects language skills in the early stages, but as it progresses, it will usually affect behavior as well.

There are two distinct types of Primary Progressive Aphasia (PPA). They are differentiated by the type of language difficulties manifested in each. In Semantic

Dementia, the patient will seem to have no difficulty speaking, but the words they are saying will make less and less sense. In Fluent Dementia, patients lose the ability to access vocabulary, and their speech will be punctuated with periods of silence as they try to recall the right word to use. People with Fluent Dementia have also been known to lose the ability to read and write.

FTD Movement Disorder

In addition to impaired language and social skills, FTD Movement Disorder is associated with two distinct movement disorders: Corticobasal Degenerative Disorder (CBD) and Progressive Supranuclear Palsy (PSP).

CBD can cause shakiness, muscle rigidity and spasms as well as a general lack of coordination. PSP will cause problems with walking, that may include frequent falls, balance and muscle stiffness. There also may develop irregular eye movements.

As with other types of dementia, it is sometimes difficult to distinguish FTD from Alzheimer's. There is no testing that can conclusively diagnose FTD, so once again any diagnosis will be clinical, based on the physician's best judgment of what is causing the symptoms being exhibited.

This may sound like stating the obvious, but it is important to never engage in self-diagnosis for this or any other form of cognitive impairment. Sometimes even very well-trained physicians struggle with forming accurate diagnoses of the different types of dementia and cognitive impairment. Leave it to the professionals. I do not know if my experience was unique, but as I have already mentioned, I did self- diagnose, and I believe I paid a heavy price for having done so. It not only delayed my treatment, but it also led to innumerable unfounded fears and prolonged the presence of extremely damaging thinking and behavior in my life.

The prognosis for FTD, as with all types of non-reversible dementia, is poor. To date, nothing has been discovered that can stop the progression of this disease. Patients will reach a state where they are bed bound and often mute.

The good news is that scientists around the globe are working to find a cure for dementia, and there is more than one lab where they believe they may have done so. There are studies currently underway all over the world searching for answers, and I am confident that soon, statistically significant evidence will be presented announcing that a way to halt this deadly disease has been found.

There is also a body of evidence showing a marked correlation between lifestyle, including diet, and the incidence of dementia. Numerous studies have been done that show there is a definite connection between diet, exercise and the maintenance or enhancement of cognitive function.

Although many currently believe there is no cure for this and other forms of dementia, HELP IS AVAILABLE for patients and the families that care for them. The Association for Frontotemporal Degeneration (AFTD) is one resource that may be reached by phone. The number in the United States is 866-507-7222.

The Alzheimer's Association, the source for much of the information in this chapter, has a 24-hour toll-free helpline that can be reached at 800-272-3900. The staff will be happy to point you to resources in your area that can provide significant types of assistance for people living with dementia and their caregivers. They can also provide a wealth of information about dementia in general. Countries all over the world have Alzheimer's associations that can be found online.

It is also well to remember that the Social Security Administration may very well be able to provide financial assistance in the form of Disability Benefits. If the illness has made gainful employment no longer possible, you may be eligible for these benefits until the age of 66, at which point you will start receiving the same benefit as if you had retired at that age.

Acknowledging the extent of the problem in the United States, the federal government recently mandated the Social Security Administration to fast-track disability claims from people with certain types of dementia. In my case, the benefits were awarded about six months after I applied. I waited so long to get any kind of help at all, from Social Security or anyone else, that I was almost ruined financially by the time I received benefits. So, one more time I am saying, based on my own experience, DO NOT DELAY IN SEEKING HELP! Help is available, but you have to ask for it.

The Mayo Clinic has an informative website at www.mayoclinic.org that contains a treasure trove of information about dementia and diseases linked to the symptoms of dementia. Among these are stroke, Huntington's disease, Parkinson's disease, and traumatic head injury as a result of either repeated trauma to the head (common among boxers, football players and unfortunately, our soldiers) or one major trauma.

Of everything that is ever written, or talked about, concerning dementia, it is almost always about Alzheimer's. Now that you have been informed about other types of dementia, I am going to provide you with a more detailed explanation of the disease so universally feared.

ALZHEIMER'S

Dozens of books have been written about Alzheimer's disease. It is not my intention here to report everything that is known about the condition, especially all the scientific minutiae about brain chemistry and biology. My intention is to present the information that I wish I had been in possession of when I was trying to deal with my own cognitive decline. This will also be of value to not only those concerned about their cognitive decline but also for those who take care of them.

The facts and figures about Alzheimer's tell a frightening story. With our nation's rapidly aging population, the cost to the country of treating and caring for people with this disease is already enormous, and it is projected to become catastrophic. Here are some of the statistics that have been gathered by the Alzheimer's Association:

- As of 2015, there were 5.4 million Americans diagnosed with Alzheimer's

- There are 30 million cases worldwide as of 2015
- Someone develops the disease every 6 or 7 seconds
- Almost two-thirds of people with Alzheimer's are women
- An estimated 25 million people were providing care for Alzheimer's patients. Some estimates are higher, and most caregivers are unpaid.
- Approximately 700,000 deaths will be caused by this disease in 2015
- It is estimated that in the year 2017 this disease, combined with all other types of dementia, cost the U.S. 259 billion dollars
- Only 45 percent of people with the disease and those who care for them have ever been given a diagnosis of Alzheimer's
- At present, there is no known cure for the disease. (Obviously, the ReCODE Protocol has changed this)

While the above statistics appear grim, there is MUCH TO BE HOPEFUL ABOUT. Many still believe the disease is always progressive and fatal. The ReCODE Protocol is now reversing symptoms of the disease in thousands of people who follow it and it is all the proof I need that this is no longer the case. Every day I wake up clear-headed and free of the constant fear that plagued me every day for many years, I know I have escaped the deadly grip of Alzheimer's.

Dr. Bredesen has formed a company, AHNP:

Precision Health, whose mission it is to make the protocol available to people everywhere. He now has approximately 1500 doctors fully trained and available to treat patients around the United States. Hopefully, there will be a specialized doctor near you soon. Currently, there are over 5000 people following the protocol, either exactly as prescribed or their own version of it. In addition, a direct to consumer set of tests are now available at www.MyCognoscopy.com.

Dozens of major universities the world over have research departments working continuously to solve the riddle of Alzheimer's. Pharmaceutical companies are testing new drugs every day that hopefully will improve conditions for people suffering from the disease. And, there are medications already available that can significantly relieve the symptoms of Alzheimer's and other forms of dementia.

There is one other fact that needs to be taken into account: Alzheimer's progresses very slowly. While still considered by many to be a fatal disease, the course of the disease can take well over a decade from beginning to end, and a lot can happen in a decade.

It is not surprising that people over the age of 55 spend more time worrying about Alzheimer's than any other disease. If you are beginning to experience memory problems, DO NOT PANIC. We now know, it is not always Alzheimer's, and, even when it is, there is hope.

Diagnosis

As we have seen, there are a number of different types

of dementia, several of them reversible, which cause symptoms similar to Alzheimer's. This makes the diagnosis of the disease difficult, but not impossible.

The investigation will begin in the doctor's office. If dementia is suspected, your doctor will take a detailed medical history. Through an examination of this history, an effort will be made to uncover other possible sources of cognitive impairment.

There are various cognitive function tests that your doctor can perform right in his office. Those tests cost nothing.

You can expect to be given blood tests to rule out vitamin deficiencies that are known to cause cognitive difficulties. It is likely tests will also be suggested to rule out interruptions to the flow of blood to the brain. PET scans are increasingly being utilized to detect evidence of Alzheimer's in the brain, but these tests may be very expensive, and insurance companies are extremely reticent to approve payment for them.

The progression of the disease has historically been tracked with a seven-stage model, each stage having its particular signs and symptoms. Dr. Barry Reisberg, Clinical Director of New York University's Aging and Dementia Research Center, has further broken some of these stages into subsets. Almost all of the information that follows comes from an article that appeared on the website www.alzinfo.org

Stage One

There are no signs of impairment of any kind during this phase. Everything appears perfectly normal, but changes are beginning to take place in the brain.

Stage Two (Normal Age Forgetfulness)

In this stage, while problems with memory and changes in thinking are just beginning, there are no observable signs of impairment. There may be signs of forgetfulness, such as a tendency to forget names or inability to remember why you have gone into a particular room, but these minor difficulties are common to a significant percentage of people as they age. Since this occurs in around 50 percent of people over the age of 65, no one has any reason to be concerned. Even close friends and family members will have no idea that anything is amiss. Recently, it has been learned, however, that people who do experience these common age-related lapses in memory are in fact, more susceptible to developing full-blown dementia as they get older.

Stage Three: Mild Cognitive Impairment

During the Mild Cognitive Impairment (MCI), there will be noticeable evidence that something isn't quite right. There will be lapses in memory that are worse than those associated with normal aging. Your family and friends would rather believe nothing is wrong and they will tell you that you're okay. However, those closest to the person may be aware something is amiss.

This refusal of friends and family to admit there is a

problem can be quite frustrating. I cannot count the number of times I was told by well-meaning friends that the changes I was experiencing were not anything to be concerned about, just part of getting older. I would have liked to believe them, but I knew at that stage, there was nothing normal about what I was experiencing.

This is also the time where things start to be frequently misplaced and increasingly difficult to find. And when found, they are often in strange places. In my case, this was an everyday occurrence. One day my telephone was eventually found in the refrigerator, on another occasion, in the clothes hamper. When I could not find something, I noticed that I became very agitated. These events seem to get the attention of the people in your life.

There may occasionally be difficulty accessing vocabulary. Random words might be exchanged for the appropriate one when speaking. One day I asked an employee to “hand me that board". There was no board there. Actually, I had wanted him to hand me a tape measure. On another occasion, I heard myself say, "This thing weighs a fortune."

An inability to plan and organize projects may begin to manifest during this period, and it may be sufficient to begin to hinder performance at work. It is not uncommon for people to start attempting to hide their problems. This becomes increasingly difficult as the disease progresses. A better strategy might be to begin to consider retirement, an excellent idea if you are in a position to do so. If retirement does not seem like an option, it is definitely time to start restructuring your responsibilities.

The beginnings of difficulties in learning new skills will arise and keeping up with innovations in technology may become increasingly challenging. There are also likely to be more frequent incidents of anxiety, often induced by minor frustrations like a lost set of keys. I did not know that when I was frantically searching for my jacket or phone.

Not everyone with MCI will experience all of these symptoms, but all of them are common. This is one of the difficulties in diagnosing the disease. The disease does not express itself in the same way in each person, and many of these symptoms are common to multiple types of dementia.

Depression, if not already present, may begin to affect the person with Alzheimer's, as their awareness of their limitations and deficits grows. They may also be conscious that they are becoming a burden. Since depression has been linked to cognitive impairment, it must be identified and treated by a health professional. If this is not done, it will not be possible to get a clear picture of the dementia. One of the hidden blessings of my illness has been the fact that I was treated for depression and while it did not end the cognitive decline, it did end the depression. I am no longer suffering from it

A large number of persons experiencing the deficits we have been discussing will never decline further, even after many years. However, the majority will, and they will begin to manifest more and more symptoms of dementia as time passes.

It was during this stage that I began to make decisions that seriously affected the well-being of my family. Had I allowed someone else to know the extent of the problems I was experiencing at this point and had I gotten some professional help, I believe the last ten years of my life would have been very different. MCI has an average duration of four to seven years.

Stage Four (Mild Alzheimer's)

In Stage Four Alzheimer's, very clear symptoms of the disease begin to manifest. A person in this phase begins to be unable to recall parts of their life history, and short-term memory worsens. Patients may not remember in the afternoon what they were doing in the morning.

The inability to manage one's own finances continues to decline, and it may become difficult to write a check correctly. It is not uncommon for people to put the wrong date and even the wrong amount on checks they do write. Remembering to sign checks can also be a problem.

During Stage Four it may become difficult to order from a menu or remember the day of the week. Towards the end of this period, people may not even remember significant recent events. They will, however, usually remember important information, such as where they live, what the weather is like outside and major current events.

In this phase of Alzheimer's, patients will

become more easily confused. They will also become increasingly prone to anxiety, often over very simple things, and new situations will occasionally frighten them. It will be increasingly obvious to everyone with whom they live and interact regularly that they are having serious problems. Close monitoring by a physician is now essential There are a number of tests that should have been conducted by now, including blood work, CT scans, MRIs, and in office neuropsychological testing to determine the extent of cognitive decline. Ideally, some of this testing should be done as soon as there are concerns. The earlier the extent of the problem is known, the better the chances for a positive outcome, and hopefully the easier it is to manage the symptoms with pharmaceuticals. While there are no existing drugs that will cure the disease, there are several that are known to improve memory. The treatment of depression and the reduction of stressors may also help to reduce symptoms.

Despite the fact that a diagnosis of Alzheimer's can be made with some certainty during this phase, many doctors are not in a hurry to do so. Since until this time Alzheimer's has been considered an incurable, fatal disease, they seem to have a reluctance to make this decision. That may explain why almost 45 percent of patients who have this illness have never been diagnosed with it. Since many now believe that the progression of Alzheimer's can be stopped, making an earlier diagnosis is even more important.

It is during this stage of the disease that subtle

changes in personality become evident. There is a lack of confidence in social situations that often manifests in a decreased desire to participate in activities that used to bring joy. Who wants to go to an art opening or a party, or anywhere they know they will run into people whose names they don't recall? Or worse, people they simply don't remember. Who wants to put themselves in any situation that exposes their weakness? I can promise you I did not.

One day I was at the local shopping center, and I ran into a young man who obviously knew me, but whose face I could not recall. I admitted I could not place him and asked him to give me a hint. He said, "How about I am the guy who house-sat for you three or four times when you were out of town a few years ago? Does that help?" Of course, I then remembered, and of course, I was totally embarrassed. After a few such experiences, it is no wonder that the desire to be out and about diminishes.

There will be a tendency to withdraw from conversation in certain settings, lest these deficits become readily observable to others. In short, there is the beginning of the desire to disengage from some of the best parts of life.

Patients will still be able to live independently while in Stage Four, but they will certainly require monitoring and assistance. This phase has an approximate duration of two years.

I believe that when I had the good fortune of learning about Dr. Bredesen's work and began my recovery from Alzheimer's, I was vacillating between stages three and four. I shall forever be grateful that the following sections about the later progression of the disease will contain nothing based on my personal journey. They will describe things I lived in fear of going through but am now confident I need not experience as long as I continue to practice the protocol.

Stage Five (Moderately Severe Decline)

Patients now will begin to need assistance with many of their day-to-day activities. People will often have difficulty in dressing themselves appropriately. It may be hard for them to choose clothing that is appropriate to the occasion or weather conditions. They may start wearing the same clothes every day. Difficulties remembering basic details about their own lives will stand in the way of independence, though they may not recognize or admit to this. Remembering their home address or even their own phone number may be impossible, and managing their finances is categorically out of the question.

It is no longer feasible for the person to be living independently. If they are living alone, it is imperative that someone has the responsibility of ensuring that proper nutrition is provided and that the basic management of the living quarters are attended to. Home care and meals-on-wheels can be useful resources at this point.

There will now be an increasing inability to recall

major events in their lives and a person may not remember in the afternoon someone that he saw in the morning. He may not remember events he has scheduled, the day of the week or what year it is.

In this period, people with Alzheimer’s need to be protected not only from themselves but also from others. Confusion is so constant, and thinking is so impaired, they are easily taken advantage of. In the present state of society, there are people whose sole occupation is preying on the elderly, and a person living alone with dementia becomes a very easy target. They should have no access to significant amounts of cash, nor the ability to attain it. In 2015, AARP Magazine reported that there have been reports of people writing hundreds of thousands of dollars in checks for home improvements that were neither necessary nor performed, and later having no recollection of having done so.

On some level, people in this phase sometimes know they are easily taken advantage of, and as a result, may become suspicious even of the people closest to them. There is a great deal of fear in the subconscious of these persons, and it often manifests as anger. People in the midst of Stage Five Alzheimer's are not always pleasant folks to be around, nor are they easy to care for. This responsibility, more often than not, falls on the shoulders of family members and loved ones. It is work, and it is arduous, and it is almost always a labor of love.

The passage through the various phases of Alzheimer's happens subtly and gradually. They can vary in duration, and they may overlap one another. On average, Stage Five has a duration of approximately one and a half years.

Stage Six (Severe Decline)

Stage Six Alzheimer's usually announces itself with the patient's inability to dress. In the fifth phase, there was difficulty choosing the right clothing, but now there is an inability to put them on without assistance. The mechanics of dressing, something they have done their entire lives, now becomes a challenge. It is not uncommon for people in Stage Six to put on a set of clothing without taking off the set they are wearing, or they may put their clothes on backward. If not supervised they may wear the same clothing day after day.

As a rule, losing the ability to dress without assistance is followed by an inability to bathe without help. And that is followed by difficulties in toileting. Patients will begin to forget to flush, and incontinence will eventually begin to be a factor. The toll on the caregiver becomes greater and greater.

During the progression of this stage, patients will begin to forget things like their children's names and may not recall what they did in their working lives. Their former life is slowly disappearing from their consciousness, and they begin to confuse who is who in their circle of relationships. At some point, they will no longer recall their own names.

It is in the sixth stage that changes in personality will become the most pronounced. Living in constant confusion, fear, and shame, they are prone to angry outbursts and may become violent. Because they are conscious of how much care they need, they may develop a fear of being left alone. It is also at this time that people may begin to wander from home and will begin to need almost constant supervision for their own safety.

The patient's ability to communicate through speech will be severely compromised at the end of this stage. Stage Six of Alzheimer's disease usually lasts less than a year and a half.

Stage Seven (Severe Alzheimer's Disease)

By now the disease has taken away almost all of the things that make life livable. Many patients will have died from natural causes by now, but for those that remain, and those who care for them, life becomes extremely difficult. Although Dr. Reisberg has further subdivided this stage into six sub-stages, for the sake of simplicity I am not going to define them.

At this point, the patient will require assistance with every function of day-to-day living. He has, or very quickly will have, lost the capacity for speech. He may have a vocabulary of five or ten words for a period of time, but as the disease progresses, he will lose even that, left only with nonverbal communication, which very well may be unclear and difficult to interpret.

The difficulty walking that may have been evidenced in Stage Six usually progresses to total immobility, most often directly after the ability to speak is gone. At the same time that the patient is losing the ability to walk unassisted, they will also be losing the capability to sit up without help. They will also tend to, while sitting, fall over if no kind of support is provided. It is possible to provide specialized chairs that provide better posture and position, and also recline.

Once speech and the ability to sit are lost, there will be an absence of facial expressions, including smiling. Rigidity in the major joints also occurs, and the patient will also lose the ability to hold their head up.

At this point, the disease will have run its course and the patient, if they have not already passed during one of the previous stages, will do so shortly. There seems to be little ability to stave off the common illnesses that occur in the elderly, and the patient will most often die as a result of one of them.

Occasionally they will pass as a result of nothing observable other than the Alzheimer's itself. The average duration of Stage Seven is approximately one and a half years.

While Dr. Reisberg has gone into much greater detail describing the symptoms and progression of the disease, I believe the information I have presented is sufficient for our needs.

Medication

At present, there are some prescription medications available that can help with managing the symptoms of the illness. While there is much debate over how well and how long these drugs work, it is a fact that many people have found long-term relief from memory loss and confusion as a result of using these pharmaceutical therapies. And, although the manufacturers of these drugs suggest that their long-term efficacy may be limited, there is anecdotal evidence that they may be helpful for many years.

The most well-known drugs available for help with dementia are a class of pharmaceuticals called cholinesterase inhibitors. They are prescribed to treat symptoms related to not only memory but to strategic thinking as well. These medicines appear to be effective for about half of the people who take them.

The first of these medications to arrive on the scene was Donepezil, commonly known as Aricept, which I began taking in late 2011 or early 2012. I am not convinced I am still benefiting from using it but I continue to do so. Once in 2016 and twice in 2017, I ran out of the medicine and missed as many as five days with no loss of cognition. I continue to take the medicine because when I first started using it I was told to never discontinue it.

It is not uncommon for some people to experience side effects from all of these drugs, but they are usually well tolerated. The most common side effects with Aricept are nausea and vomiting, loss of appetite and increasing frequency of bowel movements. I personally experienced none of these side effects.

Another side effect, one that I experienced myself, is vivid, disturbing dreams. These dreams occur in a very limited number of cases, and they will usually disappear over time. However, for the first several months when I was taking Aricept, I had horrific nightmares four or five nights a week. If there had not been so much at stake, I would have discontinued the medication, but I was not willing to do that.

In most of these dreams, I would be lost in some strange area with no telephone, no contact numbers, no money and no idea where I should go or what I should do; often in the dreams, friends would have abandoned me. Some nights I would awaken from the dream in the middle of the night and be afraid to go back to sleep for fear that the nightmares would return, which they sometimes did. It was like getting a preview of having progressed further along in the disease, and it was awful.

Another version of the dream was that I would kind of come-to in the dream after a period of several weeks of wandering and trying to find my way home. I would somehow contact a friend of my wife's, only to be told she had given up and moved out long ago.

While I am sure a psychologist could have had fun analyzing these nightmares, it was clear to me what was going on. I had deep fears about my illness, fears my conscious mind was not up to dealing with. Regardless of what their meaning was, the dreams eventually went away.

I started out on a dosage of five milligrams of Aricept once a day at bedtime. There was no change for at least a month, and then I began to find relief from my inability to access the correct words when speaking, as well as some of the confusion I had been experiencing. My memory also seemed to be in some ways better. I know my thinking was improving because it was after starting the medication that I could start to see more clearly the damage I was doing to our family's financial resources. That is my recollection although it is possible the damage was getting so bad it was undeniable.

Things seemed much improved for a few months, and I even withdrew the disability claim I had filed with the Social Security Administration. All was well for another three or four months, and then the medication seemed to stop working almost overnight. That was probably not the case, but it seemed that way. Once again, I was grasping for words and really struggling with simple tasks.

Aricept is available in three strengths: five, ten and twenty-three milligrams. I asked my Doctor to increase my dose, and he did. In the time I was waiting to see if the change would be beneficial, I reinstated my claim. A few months later the Social Security Administration sent me for an hour and a half examination with a Doctor they use for verifying eligibility. Actually, he had been tasked with debunking my application. I have been told that most are rejected on the first try. Mine was not. His diagnosis was pre-senile dementia, or Early Onset Alzheimer's. My claim was approved. Shortly after that, I began experiencing relief again, but at that point, I was convinced it would only be temporary. Today, seven years later, as a result of my experience with the Bredesen Protocol that is a moot point.

Another side-effect that I experienced with Aricept was a major loss of appetite. I lost about twenty pounds over a three or four-month period, which was fine with me as I was overweight at the time. When I later began exercising as part of the ReCODE Protocol, the weight loss became even more pronounced.

Rivastigmine, also known as Exelon, is a cholinesterase inhibitor that was approved for the treatment of mild to moderate Alzheimer's disease by the FDA in 1998. According to an article that appeared on www.medicinenet.com in July of 2015, Excelon does not produce “dramatic improvement.” It may, however, slow the progression of the symptoms. There is also clinical data showing a 25 to 30 percent improvement in memory and understanding after six months of treatment with this drug.

Excelon was granted FDA approval for the treatment of mild to moderate Alzheimer's in 2001. Like all the drugs used to treat Alzheimer's, it is not a cure for the disease. It may, however, improve memory, confusion, awareness and the ability to perform the functions of daily living.

Memantine (marketed under a number of names, the most common being Namenda) is the grand-daddy of all the drugs being used to treat Alzheimer's. It belongs to a class of drugs known as MNDA Receptor Antagonists and was first synthesized in 1968. It has been approved by the FDA for use with moderate to severe Alzheimer's. The drug appears to have no effect on patients with mild Alzheimer's but has been shown to produce a moderate decrease in clinical deterioration in more advanced stages of the disease.

Despite the relatively minimal impact Namenda has on the symptoms of the disease, according to an article on www.drugs.com in February of 2014, Namenda posted almost two billion dollars in sales in recent years. This may be due to the approval of the drug for use in cases where the patient is unable to use the cholinesterase inhibitor drugs such as Aricept.

Although the medications approved for the treatment of Alzheimer's are very limited at this time, there are new drugs being tested in labs all over the country. Some of these are looking very promising in early trials. These studies historically have involved mice. Trials with human subjects began in 2016.

The ongoing studies involving the ReCODE Protocol are providing convincing evidence that the disease can be halted, and symptoms eliminated using modalities that involve no pharmaceuticals at all. As I am writing today, it is seven years since my diagnosis of Early Onset Alzheimer's. At that time, I was showing symptoms of both stage three and stage four of the disease. If the protocol was not working, the disease should have progressed and I would be completely incapable of writing any kind of book. Instead, I sit at my computer writing these words and looking forward to having some fun this afternoon.

We have seen that Alzheimer's is a cruel disease. Over time it takes away everything that makes life meaningful and eventually it takes away life itself. While the person is hopefully not fully cognizant of all of the losses they are experiencing and perhaps spared some of the suffering, this is not true for those whose task it is to care for them.

Who is at Risk for Alzheimer's?

Researchers have been busy for years trying to determine what factors put a person at risk for developing the disease. Although 70 percent of people suffering from Mild Cognitive Impairment go on to develop advanced Alzheimer's, many do not. Science is trying to unlock the secret of why that is.

There are, however, numerous other factors that have been associated with dementia. Among them are stress, depression, medications, diet and even heredity. There is a gene, APOE 4, that has been linked to the disease and there is a website devoted to information on that subject.

It is becoming increasingly clear that there are actions you can take to reduce the likelihood of developing the disease and increasing evidence of things you can do to mitigate the symptoms of the illness should you have it.

You may want to consider participating in a clinical trial. These trials are designed to assess the efficacy of pharmaceutical and non-pharmaceutical treatments and interventions for Alzheimer’s. This is not as difficult as it may seem.

The Alzheimer's Association website www.alz.org maintains a continuously updated database that includes over two hundred ongoing trials showing promise for the treatment of Alzheimer's. On this site, you will find links to over 130 clinical trials that are enrolling new subjects as of this writing. According to the site, researchers are currently seeking 50,000 volunteers, both with and without the disease, to participate in studies.

Also, many States maintain their own websites offering support. These sites can direct you to studies that may be enrolling subjects close to your home. With so many ongoing trials, many with the potential to unlock the riddle of Alzheimer's, there is much to be hopeful about.

I hope by now I have convinced you that there are many forms of dementia, as well as forms of cognitive impairment that are in fact not dementia at all, and several that are reversible. Your family doctor, aware of your history and properly informed of your symptoms, can lead you to an eventual diagnosis, quite possibly one not nearly as devastating as what you are probably thinking.

It is now crystal clear to me that persons starting to suffer from cognitive decline are not powerless over their situation. Even if your cognition is seriously impaired, as was mine, there are many ways to improve it. There are now thousands of people who have reversed the symptom of Alzheimer's.!

AFTERWORD

It has been almost ten years since I first started having frightening incidents with my memory. It is over six years since I was diagnosed with Early Onset Alzheimer's. It is four and a half years since I moved to Mexico, hopeless and contemplating suicide.

Shortly after that move I first heard about Dr. Bredesen, finally met him, and eventually began practicing his protocol to the best of my ability. When I first heard of his work there were only nine people that had reversed the symptoms of the disease.

Today there are several thousand. In 2015, Dr. Bredesen was the only physician offering the treatment plan. He has since trained over 1500 doctors to guide people in their recovery.

Had the disease progressed untreated, I would by now be in the final stages of the illness, no longer capable of taking care of myself. Instead, I am sitting by my fireplace contemplating a joyous holiday season. I had lunch with friends today. I was not afraid I would embarrass myself or my wife. I remember everything we spoke about. I drove home without incident. It was a beautiful day. Most of my days are like that today and yours can be too. THERE IS A SOLUTION!

Made in the USA
Columbia, SC
26 January 2021

31731734R00107